P9-DBI-615

Postpartum
Depression

Postpartum Depression

Every Woman's Guide to Diagnosis, Treatment, & Prevention

SHARON L. ROAN

618.76
ROA

ADAMS MEDIA CORPORATION
Holbrook, Massachusetts

Copyright ©1997, Sharon L. Roan. All rights reserved.
This book, or parts thereof, may not be reproduced in any form without permission
from the publisher; exceptions are made for brief excerpts used in published reviews.

Published by Adams Media Corporation
260 Center Street, Holbrook, MA 02343

ISBN: 1-55850-765-5

Printed in the United States of America.

J I H G F E D C B A

Library of Congress Cataloging-in-Publication Data
Roan, Sharon L.
Postpartum depression : every woman's guide to diagnosis, treatment,
and prevention / Sharon L. Roan. — 1st ed.
p.   cm.
Includes bibliographical references and index.
ISBN 1-55850-765-5 (pbk. : alk. paper)
1. Postpartum depression—Popular works. I. Title.
RG852.R63   1997
618.7'6—dc21   97-20361
                                CIP

The writer and publisher have made every effort to secure appropriate copyright per-
missions for quotations used. Thanks are due to the following for permission to use the
material indicated:
From *The New Mothercare* by Lyn DelliQuadri and Kati Breckenridge. Copyright
©1978, Lyn DelliQuadri and Kati Breckenridge; copyright ©Lyn DelliQuadri.
From *The Birth of a Father* by Martin Greenberg. Copyright © by Martin Greenberg.
From *A Spectrum of Postpartum Adjustment* and *Babies and Jobs* by Dawn Gruen.
Copyright © by Dawn Gruen.
From *Psychopharmocology: The Fourth Generation of Progress*, Bloom and Kupfer,
eds. Copyright ©1995, Lippincott-Raven Publishers.
From *Depression After Childbirth*, 3rd Edition by Katharina Dalton. Copyright ©1996,
Oxford University Press.
From *Postpartum Psychiatric Illness: A Picture Puzzle*, Hamilton and Harberger, eds.
Copyright ©1992, University of Pennsylvania Press.

This publication is designed to provide accurate and authoritative information with
regard to the subject matter covered. It is sold with the understanding that the publisher is not engaged in rendering legal, accounting, or other professional advice. If legal
advice or other expert assistance is required, the services of a competent professional
person should be sought.
— From a *Declaration of Principles* jointly adopted by a Committee of the American
        Bar Association and a Committee of Publishers and Associations

*This book is available at quantity discounts for bulk purchases. For information,
call 1-800-872-5627 (in Massachusetts, call 617-767-8100).*

Visit our home page at http://www.adamsmedia.com

Table of Contents

Foreword

Several years ago, while working as a newspaper reporter, I was introduced to a woman unlike anyone I have ever met. She was twenty-six, waiflike, blonde, and kind. She was, and always had been, very religious. Her sentences were sprinkled with references to her religious faith. She rarely smiled. Her eyes had a kind of blank, sad look.

Sheryl Massip had been a happily married new mother when she killed her six-week-old son in 1987. Massip had become mentally ill in the few weeks following childbirth. Everyone around her noticed. No one knew quite what to do for the sleepless, weeping, paranoid young mother. Massip tried to help herself, at one point telling a doctor that she was "having a nervous breakdown." The doctor did nothing.

Massip's crime outraged the conservative community where she lived. Even her attorney at first had been reluctant to take on her case. She was tried for second-degree murder and convicted, despite a parade of mental health witnesses who testified that her actions classically fit the profile of an illness called postpartum psychosis, an illness that results in infanticide in about 3 percent of all cases.

The jurors felt sorry for her, they said. Still, they couldn't understand how Massip could have done it — killed her baby. The judge, however, had seen insanity before. And, a few days before Christmas in 1988, he reversed the jury's ruling and set Massip free as long as she continued to receive psychiatric care.

When I interviewed her a few months later, she was relieved and yet destroyed. As I got to know her over the course of several interviews, I became convinced that this woman had not willfully killed her child, just as she had not willfully become mentally ill. It angered me that the jury, who heard the scientific evidence, had not understood this mental disorder. And as I explored the scientific research on postpartum disorders, I was stunned to find out that although Massip's illness, postpartum psychosis, is very rare, a great many women suffer serious mood disorders after childbirth. Most studies estimate that 10 percent of new mothers become clinically depressed in the postpartum period. Many more suffer postpartum blues, and some experience anxiety or obsessive disorders.

Sheryl Massip's experience is one of two reasons why I decided to write this book. The other reason involves three women named Hope, Maggie, and Nancy. A few years ago we all lived in the same neighborhood and were the mothers of young children. Although we were scattered over several blocks, we bonded together. We arranged play dates for our kids, had parties, and listened to each other's complaints about our old, dilapidated houses.

As I got to know these remarkable women, I was intrigued to find out that postpartum illness was no stranger to my own neighborhood. I had not experienced the illness, although I well understood the adjustment problems and stresses of the postpartum period acutely, because both my children had health problems after their births. My friend Hope also struggled against the stress of combining motherhood with career and dealing with babies with ear infections. Nancy and Maggie each drew a worse lot. Maggie suffered from depression that was difficult to treat. And Nancy, following the birth of her second child, was overcome by a severe postpartum depression that required hospitalization; it shattered her life and the lives of her husband and children for months. Fortunately, she recovered, as did Maggie.

The rate of postpartum illness in my own small social circle of four women was a whopping 50 percent. I became convinced that too little is known about this issue and far too little is said about it. There have been many advances in women's health care in the past decade that have raised awareness on such issues as premenstrual syndrome, osteoporosis, heart disease, and breast cancer. However, not enough women of childbearing age realize it is during the postpartum period that they are at highest risk for mental illness and that a pattern of lifelong recurrent bouts of depression is most likely to begin.

Thus, it is to Sheryl, Maggie, Nancy, and the fifty or so other women whom I interviewed for this book that I owe a debt of thanks. Their experiences enlightened me. And I fervently hope my journalistic efforts in the pages that follow will enlighten others.

I also owe profound thanks to the many health professionals whose research and words of wisdom are reported on here. And finally, I wish to express a heartfelt thank-you to my friend Suzi Bruno; my agent, Julie Castiglia; my editor, Anne Weaver; and my husband, Michael Lednovich, for their support.

Sharon L. Roan
September 24, 1996
Orange, California

CHAPTER ONE

Recognizing Postpartum Depression

For many women, pregnancy is one of the happiest times of their lives. Some women nurture dreams from their childhoods about having a baby. Couples sometimes try for many months or years to become pregnant, and they feel as if they have been granted life's greatest blessing when the baby is finally on the way. Most couples view a child as a sign of love and deep commitment between them. The child represents a future of sharing, of creating traditions and memories; a child will carry the family name and heritage into the future. From this standpoint, it doesn't seem surprising that, statistically, pregnant women are at a very low risk for experiencing depression and related mood disorders. And, given such longing for a child, it might be expected that the period after having a baby would also be fulfilling and joyous. But for too many women, the happiness, contentment, and excitement of the prenatal period dissolves into baffling feelings of sadness and anxiety — or worse — after the baby is born.

> *Four years ago, I was pregnant and feeling happy and excited. I had never heard the term* postpartum depression. *By the time I went into labor I was barely familiar with the term. I read a lot. In fact, my answer to everything is to go find a book on the subject. So when I was expecting, I read books on child-*

birth, books on pregnancy, and books on infant care. And the most any of these books had to say about postpartum depression was that "some women feel blue a few days after the birth of a baby . . . they become weepy . . . it goes away." Three weeks later I was living a nightmare. Everything was too big for me to cope with.

Postpartum psychiatric illness encompasses a range of syndromes and disorders from a mild feeling of blues that lasts just a few days to serious, long-lasting clinical depression. During the postpartum period (generally defined as the year following childbirth), women are more vulnerable to depression than at any other time in their lives.

The statistics are sobering. About 10 to 20 percent of women develop depression, panic disorder, or some form of psychiatric illness after the birth of a child. More women are admitted to psychiatric hospitals during the first two months following childbirth than at any other time period. According to one study, women in their childbearing years were four times more likely to experience a major depression than women not in their childbearing years.[1]

After a woman has had a child, the risk of developing a mental illness never drops back to its prepregnancy level. One study estimated the rate of serious psychiatric illness to be twenty times greater after a woman has borne a child.[2] This observation is striking when you consider that people who suffer from the loss of a loved one, a divorce, or the loss of a business — typical stressful life events — are about two to seven times more likely to suffer from a serious depression. So, having a baby is a riskier event than any of these. Motherhood is truly hazardous to your health.

One of the most mystifying aspects of postpartum illness is that it strikes unsuspecting families. The majority of women who become ill have never been clinically depressed or even received psychological counseling. About 70 percent of women admitted to psychiatric units in the postpartum period have no history of mental disorders.[3] They are often high-achieving, well-adjusted women who have planned their pregnancies and are eagerly looking forward to motherhood. They rejoice in childbirth and love their babies. So, the onset of depression, anxiety, or psychosis is the last thing they expect. As one mother put it, "I think I handled the death of my beloved father better than the births of my two children!"

It is no wonder women's expectations often clash with reality. Society has long portrayed motherhood in a way that few women today would recognize as legitimate. The traditional image of motherhood is one of fulfillment and bliss; and the image of the mother herself is saintlike, calm, and utterly competent. What we have failed to admit is that motherhood is tough. And the demands of the role, combined with physical factors, cultural forces, and other life problems, erodes the mental health of many women. If you are one such mother, the most reassuring fact about postpartum illness is that it can almost always be successfully treated. You, your infant, and your family will recover from the turmoil. And the very reasons that you had a baby will once again seem clear, as these new mothers who have recovered from postpartum illness have discovered:

> *Last night while I was feeding her she swung her little hand up to my lips and held her fingers there. I kissed her fingers and she began to smile behind her bottle. We played this little game for the rest of the feeding. I wouldn't trade moments like that for anything.*

> • • •

> *When I look at my husband now I am filled with a sense of thankfulness and love for him. I can't believe how strong and loving he was during my awful depression. He saved my life. We are much closer now than we were before. Our marriage has*

a strength that we earned by surviving a very tough time.

Depression

To better understand how a vital, young mother can become handicapped by a postpartum illness, it is helpful to learn a little about depression in general. It's typical to have bad days, to feel sad occasionally, even for several days. But depression is more than that. It is marked by the loss of happiness or pleasure and a feeling of emptiness. These are words from one new mother experiencing a rather severe postpartum depression, but she speaks for many depressed people:

> *Days that were supposed to be filled with joy quickly turned into pain and isolation for myself and my husband. I felt trapped in a world of hopelessness and despair. I was immobilized and couldn't perform the simplest tasks that were routine before. I was a zombie who literally had not slept for days. My only recollection of that time are fragments of a puzzle, as constant confusion took over my mind. I experienced racing thoughts and delusional thinking.*

Depression affects an individual physically and dramatically alters one's feelings, thoughts, and behavior. It doesn't just lift as the situation improves. One 1989 study found that the poor functioning — the general inability to cope with life — caused by depression was as severe or worse than that associated with eight major chronic medical conditions including hypertension, diabetes, and arthritis.[4] "Depression is often misunderstood. It is not a passing mood. It is not a personal weakness. Depression is a major health disorder," declared authorities in a recent National Institute of Mental Health report.[5]

It's easy to blame depression on personal weaknesses or even the state of one's soul. Current research links the illness to neurochemical changes in the brain. In general, two types of depression are described: endogenous and reactive. Endogenous means its underlying cause is probably a biochemical imbalance in the brain. Reactive means it is transient and caused by stress, negative thought patterns, or lifestyle changes, such as the depression someone can experience when going through a divorce.

Some people may be genetically vulnerable to depression. Under this hypothesis, susceptible people first experience the illness when they undergo severe stress. Symptoms of the illness, such as insomnia and poor appetite, may cause changes in the brain — what researchers call a "kindling effect" — making that person more vulnerable to further episodes of depression. After repeated bouts, the body may lapse into depression on its own without a stressful event triggering it. In other words, the initial illness leaves an imprint on the person's neurochemistry.

Since depression can become chronic, it's important to identify and treat the illness as early as possible to prevent recurrences. Yet, only one in three depressed people seeks treatment, and some who seek help do not get the appropriate therapy, which typically includes antidepressants, psychotherapy, and family counseling, or some combination of these. The illness doesn't always progress from mild symptoms to more severe ones, but left untreated, it usually lasts about a year. Symptoms can range and vary depending on the factors that caused it. Depression is sometimes compared with arthritis in that it can be a chronic problem that varies in kind and causality. Like other chronic conditions, depression can be managed with an arsenal of treatments and behavioral changes.

WOMEN AND DEPRESSION

For women, depression and its related disorders are of special concern. "Depression was and is one of the most serious mental health problems of the '80s and '90s," report the authors of the 1990 book *Women and Depression* by the American Psychological Association

National Task Force on Women and Depression. "Women's risk for depression exceeds that of men by two-to-one. This is one of the most consistent findings in the research literature and occurs throughout many different countries and ethnic groups."

One of every four women will have a serious clinical depression at some time in her life. It usually strikes women in their prime, between the ages of twenty-five to forty-four, the years of bearing and raising children. At any one time, at least seven million American women have diagnosable depression.

The reproductive cycle appears to be of key importance in explaining why women are so highly vulnerable to depression. For instance, about half of all women experience some mood disturbance around the time of menstruation, and women who experience premenstrual syndrome (PMS) are at increased risk of developing postpartum depression.

Mood disorders are also somewhat more prevalent among women who have had hysterectomies or are going through menopause. But social, economic, and emotional factors are believed to play a role in the onset of depression as well. For that reason, many experts contend that physiology, lifestyle, personality, and the way society treats women must all be considered possible causes for the higher rates of depression in women.

Although great strides have been made in understanding depression in general, little is known about how depression in women differs from that in men. Some theories suggest that women's traditional role as caretakers heightens stress and the risk of depression. Other studies have noted that while men may respond to bad moods by engaging in physical activities or events that distract them from their feelings, women are more likely to ruminate over their feelings — a response that tends to amplify the sadness.

POSTPARTUM ILLNESS

Risk factors for postpartum illness, like those for depression, can be biological (hormonal and genetic), social, or cognitive. They can also be based on personality and lifestyle. Postpartum illness does not discriminate between different races, socioeconomic groups, or personalities. However, certain cultures seem immune from the disorder, perhaps due to social customs that emphasize nurturing the new mother.

There are a bewildering range of factors that might increase the risk of experiencing a postpartum illness. But even women who have not had a postpartum illness can identify with several of these descriptors, some of which contradict each other. For instance, you may be more vulnerable if you are a first-time mother or have several children, or if you are a very young or a much older mother. In addition, you may be more vulnerable if you have had a long interval or a very short interval between pregnancies, or if you have a personal or family history of mental illness or no such history.

Other risk factors include:

- Past experience of physical, emotional, or sexual abuse
- Stress during pregnancy or at the time of delivery
- Overanxiousness and the inability to cope with change
- Conflicting feelings about becoming a mother
- Unrealistic expectations of motherhood
- Lack of preparation for motherhood
- Marriage strain
- A poor relationship with your own mother
- Lack of support and help from others
- Social isolation
- A sick or colicky infant
- Stressful life events (such as moving, money problems, or a death in the family)

What you can see from this broad list is that postpartum illness can arise from many different but stressful life situations — emotional as well as physical. The only obstetric-related variables that correlate with postpartum depression are giving birth prematurely or giving birth to twins, says one expert on the disorder, Dr. Douglas Bright. The patient's mood during pregnancy seems to have little to do with the mood afterward. "In fact, women who are depressed during pregnancy generally are not the ones who have depression after delivery," he says. After birth, the strongest predictive factors of the illness are the lack of support from the spouse and difficulties in the marriage.

Definitions of postpartum psychiatric illness are usually divided into three types or degrees of severity: blues, depression, and psychosis. However, the illness may encompass much more than that. Many experts now refer to a "spectrum" of illnesses or a collection of disorders that may even overlap. Nevertheless, most doctors and therapists find it helpful to divide the disorders into classifications that include maternal blues, major postpartum depression (which can range from mild to moderate to severe), postpartum psychosis, obsessive-compulsive disorder occurring in the postpartum period, and panic disorder.

POSTPARTUM BLUES

It was 4 A.M., and Carolyn sat in the darkness in her infant son's room in the hand-carved rocking chair she had purchased with so much happiness just two months before. She remembered that day clearly. She had taken the day off from work to enjoy a shopping spree to purchase all the lovely things that her first child would need — and that she would need in order to be a good mother to him. She had roamed dreamily through the store running her hand over the smooth, curved wood rockers before selecting this wide, comfortable chair. She had envisioned the happiness she would feel, cuddling her child to her as they rocked and sang, his little eyes staring into her face.

She wondered what had become of her dream. As she sat in the chair, nursing her irritable child for the third time since 10 P.M., tears rolled down her cheeks. She was exhausted. She felt weak. She abhorred the resentment and anger she had felt when she heard the child crying again to be fed. She hated her husband for sleeping, for being able to escape to work in the morning. She made a mental note to herself that she must call her pediatrician in the morning to ask if she should start giving the baby a bottle. She was convinced he was not getting enough of her breastmilk. She had been at home with her son for two weeks. In four more weeks, she would have to return to work. Why wasn't this period she had looked forward to turning out like she had expected?

The term *baby blues* sounds mild and unthreatening, but the new mother who is experiencing it often has feelings that are very intense. It is, however, a temporary phenomenon that has no long-term effects on either the mother or baby.

Baby blues, or maternity blues, is a period of sadness experienced by an estimated 70 to 80 percent of all new mothers in the first days or weeks following childbirth.[6] In Great Britain, the syndrome has been called the three-, four-, or five-day blues or the "10-day weepies," which represents the time of onset or about how long the episode lasts, says Dr. Katharina Dalton, a British physician and expert on mood disorders and the reproductive cycle. Normally, blues will strike on the third or fourth day postpartum and will last no longer than two weeks.

The tendency to burst into tears often and for little reason is characteristic of maternity blues. Rapid mood swings are common as well as insomnia, exhaustion, and some confusion. If you have the blues, you may have trouble concentrating and feel as if your thinking is muddled. You might feel anxious, irritable, and even hostile toward others, most likely your husband! You might feel isolated and lonely.

My husband only stayed home with me for two days. Then I was on my own with the baby. I was overwhelmed by everything I had to do. I was in tears by noon. People would call and I would take a deep breath and tell them I was fine. But I really felt very much alone.

Some experts suggest "the blues" is actually a time of heightened emotions — both positive and negative — for new parents. One study found that the first few weeks postpartum are unique because of the fluctuation of moods in general, not necessarily because depressive moods are more common.[7] The parents commonly endure moods associated with anxiety and concern over their ability to cope; but they also experience great happiness. However, they generally describe themselves as less energetic and more tearful.

Difficulties in the postpartum period appear to fit what psychologist Ellen McGrath, an expert on depression and the author of *When Feeling Bad Is Good*, calls "realistic bad feelings" that often arise from "contemporary female experiences." "It's normal for negative or difficult experiences to produce sadness, pain, and disappointment. Bad feelings can be good because they teach us the most important life lessons and inspire and motivate us to grow." Certainly, becoming a mother is a major life change that requires such growth.

There is also a physical component to postpartum blues. The likelihood that blues will peak on the third to fifth day suggests a biological cause, such as the rapid decline of hormones that occurs as a woman's body adjusts from a pregnant to a nonpregnant state. But there is no solid evidence linking particular hormones and moods to support this theory. And experts and mothers note that stresses common during this period, such as a crying infant, learning to breastfeed, and lack of sleep, contribute heavily.

In short, maternity blues is short-lived and can be treated with education, support, reassurance, and rest. It does not require treatment with antidepressants or sleeping medications.

Maternity blues wouldn't be as difficult if couples were prepared for it. This preparation could take place in childbirth education classes or be included in postpartum instructions when you leave the hospital with the baby. Couples in childbirth education classes should ask about postpartum illness if the subject is not mentioned. Moreover, when you leave the hospital with a new baby, you should receive information from a doctor or nurse on symptoms of the blues and depression and when to call for help.

Even if you feel you "only" have the blues, a much more serious postpartum illness — psychosis — often begins with symptoms that resemble the blues. In the past, there have been cases in which women gravely ill with postpartum psychosis have been mislabeled as suffering from the blues. If you have any symptoms of the blues that persist one month or longer after childbirth or that seem to be getting progressively worse, you should see a competent physician. A physician who dismisses your concerns without hearing them out is not a competent physician. Information on how to find a good doctor or therapist will be presented in a later chapter.

Women often ask, "How do you know when the blues has become something more?" The answer is to ask for help if you are not sure. Do not be embarrassed to seek support and reassurance in coping with your feelings, even those you think are "just the blues." You can also use this rule of thumb: If the symptoms gradually diminish as your "problems" seem to subside, you've probably been experiencing either the blues or what is called an "adjustment disorder," the period of time when you are getting used to a major change in your life — a new baby.

POSTPARTUM DEPRESSION

Postpartum depression is astonishingly common and yet is the most complicated and least understood of all the psychiatric disorders that occur in the immediate period after childbirth. At least 10 percent of all new mothers experience postpartum depression — about

300,000 women each year in the United States. The number who actually seek treatment is far less than that; and less than a few hundred each year are hospitalized.[8]

Postpartum depression can be mild, moderate, or severe enough to include suicidal thoughts and require hospitalization. Its onset can be gradual and insidious or sudden, but it often occurs within two to four weeks after childbirth. For some women, it begins as the blues but lingers and develops into a serious condition.

> *I'd get the kids to day care and would drive around*
> *on my sales job. I'd have a hard time facing people.*
> *I'd see two people a day instead of seeing twenty.*
> *Eventually, I started taking the kids to day care and*
> *would just go home.*

Although postpartum depression might be mild and short-lived (a matter of weeks), vanishing on its own, the most common pattern is for the syndrome (if left untreated) to languish for several months or a year. For some mothers it can cause changes in personality and lifestyle and persist throughout life.

Some women continue to cope and remain functional, even though they feel awful; others are virtually bedridden. Sometimes there is an obvious cause, such as giving birth to a child with severe health problems. But more often, the cause is obscure or multifactorial.

Postpartum depression consists of many of the same symptoms as the blues but with increasing severity, frequency, and extremity, experts say. The signs and symptoms to look for are:

- Rapid mood swings
- Dramatic changes in sleep patterns, such as insomnia, or the need for constant sleep with continual feeling of fatigue
- A serious inability to concentrate characterized by muddled thinking and fogginess; or "frenetic zooming," the feeling of your mind racing, or memory loss

- Numbness, a lack of interest in your world, activities, and other people; a sense of hopelessness and despair; lack of interest in sex; inability to cope
- Irritability or explosive temper; feeling out of control
- Obsessive thoughts, usually about your infant, such as repeated visions of the infant falling from its cradle; irrational fears about your baby's health
- Physical ailments such as body aches, dry skin, cold extremities, hair loss, weakness, loss of energy, palpitations, difficulty with breastfeeding, constipation, swelling of hands and feet, and headaches; exaggerated changes in appetite, often the inability to eat
- Thoughts of dying or suicidal thoughts, self-deprecatory thoughts, thoughts of hurting your baby, other scary or bizarre thoughts
- Anxiety, panicky feelings, or actual panic attacks
- Feeling overwhelmed with sadness and emotion
- Anger or ambivalence about your baby
- Isolation
- Feelings of guilt or shame that you're not a good mother
- Unusual new fears or phobias
- Hallucinations

> *I remained functional the whole time. It was extremely difficult. I could not concentrate. I could not read. I would read the same line over and over. I had this feeling of immobility. But I carried on. I picked up my boy. I did the grocery shopping.*

Postpartum illness is difficult to distinguish in part because some of the classic depressive symptoms, such as sleep disturbance, decrease in sexual interest, and appetite changes, are the norm for most postpartum women. But there are some significant symptoms that appear to be unique to postpartum depression and represent something more than the usual psychological and physical stresses associated with this period. These include:

- Worsening of sleep disturbances and insomnia despite deep fatigue
- Eating problems
- Increasing intensity of depression or irritability, particularly if these feelings are unrelated to events (this symptom often manifests itself in self-deprecatory thoughts, such as: "I'm a terrible mother. Why did I think I could take care of a baby?")
- Inability to counteract the symptoms by asking for help or taking a nap
- Withdrawal and isolation, even from your spouse
- Misinterpretation of the baby's needs and cues, such as not responding to the baby's cries or worrying excessively about the baby's health

Another clue associated with postpartum illness is the dramatic change of moods. Dr. James Hamilton, a leading expert on postpartum psychiatric illness in the United States, first described the mercurial nature of a depressed new mother's mood swings as "a tendency for very rapid and unpredictable changes to occur. Patients may move from apparent lucidity to confusion and delirium, then express bizarre delusional ideas. They may be hyperactive and euphoric and then quickly sink to a mood of deep depression. Between psychotic syndromes patients may appear to be quite rational."

Other experts, meanwhile, attach great significance to the symptom of irritability and its relationship to premenstrual irritability. Katharina suggests that women who suffer from premenstrual tension syndrome are at higher risk for postpartum depression because of sensitivity to the hormonal fluctuations that trigger both.

I think I first noticed something was wrong with my wife when friends brought dinner over and she kind of tossed them out of the house. Their five-year-old was running around the house and it seemed to upset Rose. I had to tell our friends, "Hey, it's not your kid. Rose is just not herself." This was about five days after the birth. She began writing little Post-it notes and pasting them all over the kitchen counter. I told the guys at work about her and they said that she was going through a lot and to give her a break. The next night I knew something was really wrong. She fed the baby for a few minutes and then handed the baby to me and said. "Get the baby away."

• • •

I used to feel beautiful. I used to feel sexy, attractive. All that is gone. My body never went back to its shape, even though I lost all the weight. I feel dowdy and frumpy and very unsexual. I feel like all I am — my whole purpose — is just to be a maid and a cow.

Although many women expect to feel tired and disorganized after having a baby, they also expect "to feel good about themselves, their babies, and families. For many women this is not the case," said one expert. From being competent women, they feel as if they have become "inadequate helpless people." They remember themselves as successful and in control and feel they have misplaced that identity since having a baby. The new mother may subsequently feel inadequate, helpless, like a failure, incompetent, or foolish.

I had a terrible fear of being alone. I didn't fear I would do anything to the baby. But I was so dizzy. I was afraid I would pass out and worried about what would happen to the baby. I was afraid I would drop the baby.

"The mental confusion poses a problem and makes women frightened of going out, afraid that they will hand out the wrong fares on the buses, or absent-mindedly walk out of a shop without paying," Dalton says. These women become frightened of themselves and their own actions because "they cannot understand what is going on within them." It is not uncommon for a woman to dread her husband's leaving in the morning or to beg him to stay home from work.

> *My mind left my body a couple of times. You're not getting any sleep and you're always trying to think one step ahead about what the baby needs. My husband would tell me something and I would have no recollection of the conversation.*

Some milder forms of postpartum depression vanish on their own, but if you have symptoms that are frequent, continuous, or more intense, that is the signal that you need professional help. The treatment for postpartum depression varies widely according to its cause and severity. Sometimes counseling alone is adequate. Other times, medication or even hospitalization is required. There are many good alternatives and options. Any treatment you undergo, however, should include education and support for both you and your family.

POSTPARTUM PSYCHOSIS

Postpartum psychosis is a bizarre and unusual disorder, occurring in just one or two among one thousand births. If psychosis occurs, it usually begins shortly after childbirth, from day three to day fourteen, with rapidly changing symptoms common to postpartum blues and depression. But the symptoms will greatly intensify to include agitation, delusions, hallucinations, delirium, or mania.

A psychotic mother often refuses to eat and is hyperactive. Other symptoms include inability to sleep, suspiciousness, and nonsensical talk. Dreams may become confused with reality. Some mothers say they hear their babies crying even when they are not with them. Thoughts of suicide and infanticide are common. A psychotic mother can have periods of calm and appear to be quite sane. But because of the risks involved, and the rapidity in which a woman's condition can change and deteriorate, postpartum psychosis should be treated as a medical emergency that requires immediate hospitalization.

Because of its rapid onset and its incidence in women who have no history of mental illness, many experts believe changing hormones play a significant role in the development of postpartum psychosis. Fortunately, the disorder is usually successfully treated and generally lasts only a few days or weeks. Women who have psychosis, however, commonly lapse into a postpartum depression that can be long lasting if they do not receive appropriate treatment. Some experts define this as a separate illness called "postpartum psychotic depression." These patients, especially, may appear normal at times, misleading doctors to overlook the risk of violent behavior.

OBSESSIVE-COMPULSIVE DISORDER AND PANIC DISORDER

Scientists have recently discovered that two other well-known mental health disorders can occur for the first time in the postpartum period: obsessive-compulsive disorder (OCD) and panic disorder. Like depression and psychosis, these disorders can be very successfully treated.

People with OCD have repeated, uncontrollable thoughts and may feel forced to act out meaningless behaviors repeatedly, such as washing their hands and cleaning. The behavior appears to rest on the desire to be in control or the fear of making a mistake or harming another person. In postpartum women, obsessive thoughts usually begin to occur about two to six weeks after childbirth. These thoughts can involve killing or harming the baby. The thoughts are conscious and usually intensify, and the mother may eventually start to avoid being with her baby. Fortunately, the new mother with OCD rarely acts out her obsessive ruminations.

Panic disorder can also emerge for the first time during pregnancy or the postpartum period. Someone with this disorder feels extremely anxious and can have shortness of breath, chest pain, and feelings of terror or impending doom. The new mother with panic disorder may or may not have depression, but if she does, it is usually less prominent than the symptoms of panic.

Panic disorder is common among women of childbearing age and is twice as common among women as among men. The emergence of the disorder for the first time in the postpartum period could be coincidental, but stressful life events can precipitate panic attacks. Childbirth, although considered a positive event by most people, is stressful. If a woman has a vulnerability to this disorder, the postpartum period, with its many stressors, may trigger its onset. Moreover, some research suggests panic disorder is triggered by the female hormone progesterone. During pregnancy, progesterone levels are about 170 times higher than before pregnancy.

Scientists have also discovered that depressive disorders, panic disorder, and OCD may share some similarities in the ways they are triggered in the brain and in the kinds of pharmacological agents they respond to. This could be more evidence that each of these disorders in the postpartum period may be influenced by an imbalance in the body's neurochemistry as a result of shifting hormones.

THE PROBLEM WITH DEFINITIONS

Unfortunately, none of these descriptions of postpartum blues, depression, psychosis, obsessive-compulsive disorder, or panic disorder fit neatly with individual reality. Many cases overlap various syndromes, or change from one to another. Diagnosis may not be obvious. The line between what is normal and abnormal is occasionally even debatable.

However, you should regard the blues as well as more serious disorders as important, because they all, to some extent, change your behavior, personality, and outlook. Too often, Hamilton points out, family members will bemoan that "she has never been the same since the birth of her last child." Medical experts should know that the postpartum period is one of high risk for mental illness. You and your family may have to be persistent in finding the right professional for help.

Don't be thrown off track if medical professionals disagree or even put different "names" on your condition. Even when a problem is identified, doctors and therapists sometimes disagree over what name to call it. Medical records show postpartum illness is occasionally called schizophrenia, atypical psychosis, bipolar disorder, depression, organic mental disorder or postpartum depression, postnatal depression, or puerperal illness. No wonder new mothers and their families are unsure about their conditions!

For you and your family, the important point is not what your illness is called; it's whether you are getting support and are recovering. Is your physician or therapist listening to you and your family? Does the professional have a clear treatment plan? Does this individual or health care team seem familiar with postpartum illness? If you feel uncomfortable about your care in any way, don't hesitate to turn to another health professional.

When a postpartum disorder disrupts the road between conception and your visions of happiness with your family, there is much to know, learn, and understand. Society's idealized notions of motherhood have, for a long time, led to a silencing of the voices of women who recognized that reality is sometimes quite different. As such, until very recently, women with postpartum psychiatric illness suffered without the benefit of medical care, misunderstood by their husbands, parents, friends, and doctors.

But today there are many more competent obstetricians, nurses, social workers, psychiatrists, and psychologists who know how to prevent, recognize, and treat postpartum disorders. Also, many new mothers and their spouses are speaking out about the disorder and counseling other parents. Help is available, and you can find it.

CHAPTER TWO

Making the Diagnosis

A fter recognizing a postpartum disorder, the next step to recovery is finding the right people to help you. If you are experiencing maternity blues, often all that you'll need is loving, family support. But if you are experiencing anxiety, panic, or depression, you may need professional help. There is much that can be done to help you heal, although it may be difficult to get started on the road to recovery. Sometimes doctors can be barriers to successful treatment. Even the new mother or her family can inadvertently make matters worse. Let's look at how to deal with both of those situations.

WHAT DOCTORS THINK ABOUT POSTPARTUM ILLNESS

It is impossible to estimate just how many new mothers have postpartum depression because many women are never diagnosed and treated. The disorder isn't recognized because some doctors simply don't believe it exists. Doctors generally acknowledge that some women become sad, depressed, anxious, or psychotic in the weeks and months following childbirth, but some medical professionals also contend that postpartum illness is no different from a psychiatric disorder experienced at any other time of life. To these doctors, a major depression suffered by a woman in her late fifties is no different than that of a twenty-five-year-old woman with a seven-week-old child. Some physicians have even suggested that postpartum depression is no different from the blueslike syndrome that occurs in many patients postoperatively. Postoperative blues is thought to be a reaction to acute physical stress.

But because psychiatric illnesses occur so much more commonly during the first month after childbirth, other physicians are convinced that postpartum disorders are distinctly different than psychiatric disorders occurring at other times of life. Dr. James Hamilton, an expert in the field, is the father of the theory that postpartum illness emerges as a result of physiological changes brought on by pregnancy, childbirth, and the return to a nonpregnant state. No one understands completely how these physical changes relate to mood, but enough is known to assume that postpartum illness has biological underpinnings. Although social and psychological factors should not be ignored, Hamilton says these are secondary to the biological trigger. These biological changes are imbalances in the endocrine system (the system that controls hormones) as the woman's body adjusts from a pregnant to a nonpregnant state. Not everyone agrees that physiological components always contribute to postpartum illness; however, it is because of pioneers like Hamilton that postpartum illness is receiving more recognition as a mental health problem deserving special attention.

Experts have also noted that there are particular symptoms that occur commonly among women experiencing postpartum illness that do not typically occur among other psychiatric patients. These include:

- Eating problems
- Depressed feelings of greater intensity and longer duration
- Inability to counteract fatigue
- Withdrawal and social isolation
- Poor interaction with the baby
- Rapidly changing symptoms

Other characteristics of postpartum illness that set it apart from general psychiatric illness include:

- A tendency to relapse after subsequent births
- Delirium, confusion, and hallucination, which are relatively rare in other types of depression and psychosis
- No history of mental illness
- Few problems that typically lead to depression, such as problems with relationships or finances

> *I was the last person you would expect to have postpartum depression. My husband and I both come from large, loving families. We had a solid marriage and wanted a baby. We tried for almost two years before I became pregnant. We were ecstatic. I was the typical, beaming mother-to-be. But within two weeks after having the baby, I felt like I wanted to die. My anxiety was so overwhelming I couldn't leave the house. My heart beat so fast at times I thought I was having a heart attack. I stood by the baby's crib, guarding him. After awhile, everything became a blur. I didn't know what was real and what wasn't.*

A HISTORY OF POSTPARTUM ILLNESS

There is no hard proof that postpartum illness is unique from other mental health disorders. Even so, postpartum disorders should be considered distinct disorders for various reasons. For example, nontraditional treatment may be given for postpartum depression. Factors such as breastfeeding and sleep deprivation must be taken into consideration when prescribing medications to new mothers. Moreover, the special consequences of depression should be considered in a new mother's treatment. For example, her relationship with her baby should be nurtured while she is recovering, and her family (husband, other children, extended family members) should also be given support.

The idea that postpartum psychiatric disorders have distinct causes and consequences is not new. Postpartum psychosis was described by Hippocrates in the fourth century B.C. as a severe case of insomnia and restlessness that began on the sixth day in a woman who bore twins. The first meaningful scrutiny of postpartum disorders took place during the nineteenth century. In 1858, French physician Louis Victor Marce studied and wrote about postpartum psychiatric illness. Marce noted melancholy, anemia, weight loss, constipation, and menstrual abnormalities. He also described confusion, faulty memory, and fogginess — now recognized as hallmark symptoms in postpartum illness.

But disagreement over the disorder began in the twentieth century, when some physicians initiated efforts to give all psychiatric ailments names and definitions that would be agreed upon worldwide. Although this effort would seem to be helpful, the leaders of this reform proceeded to remove the words *postpartum, puerperal* and *postnatal* from the psychiatric dictionary. Thus, the first edition of the *Diagnostic and Statistical Manual of Mental Disorders (DSM)* — a kind of "bible" for doctors that describes all known psychiatric disorders and how to treat them — was published by the powerful American Psychiatric Association in 1952 without any mention of childbearing and its relationship to psychiatric illness. This omission continued until very recently and is a major reason why postpartum illness has been under-recognized. According to Hamilton, "the vast majority of physicians believed that if the name of an illness were removed, this meant that the illness did not exist."

WHY POSTPARTUM ILLNESS CAN BE HARD TO DIAGNOSE

The decision to exclude all mention of the postpartum period held up through several subsequent editions of the DSM. And with the connection between childbirth and mental illness ignored in the DSM, research on postpartum psychiatric disorders fell off until the 1980s.

In 1980, however, Dr. Ian Brockington of Great Britain (where postpartum psychiatric illness has been much more accepted and researched) held an international meeting on postpartum illness. The physicians who attended this landmark event founded the Marce Society, a group of professionals dedicated to advancing the understanding and treatment of postpartum psychiatric illness.

But the formation of this small society did not offset the confusion that has resulted from the omission of the link between childbirth and mental illness in the DSM. The third revision of the text, the DSM-III, published in 1980, states that "there is no compelling evidence that postpartum psychosis is a distinct entity." Another revision, published in 1987, was generally heralded for its improvements over past editions because it contained more detailed definitions and information. But its only mention of postpartum illness is to practically dismiss it because of its complexity.

The latest revision, DSM-IV, published in 1994, was preceded by an intense discussion on the topic of postpartum illness, but again excludes postpartum depression, psychosis, anxiety, or any of the other observed variations as separate and distinct illnesses. Although many health professionals and women considered this omission disappointing, DSM-IV does contain a few additions that may help in the recognition and diagnosis of postpartum disorders.

In addition, the DSM-IV warns doctors of the risks of suicide and infanticide in severe cases of psychosis, of the risk of recurrence in subsequent pregnancies, and that the healthy development of the mother-infant relationship is dependent upon prompt treatment. However, the DSM-IV does not answer critical questions about postpartum illness, for example, what causes it?

POSSIBLE CAUSES

At this point, you may be wondering if anyone knows anything about postpartum illness. But much *is* known.

> *I was aware of postpartum depression and decided to give myself a week to try and snap out of it. When it didn't happen, I knew I needed to get some professional help and I did. I gradually improved, and when my daughter was nine months old, I felt I could take over all my responsibilities. As my daughter's first birthday approached, I was afraid that bad memories would return and I would sink back into a depression. But that didn't happen. We've grown very close and I feel that I've developed parenting skills that I never had before. While I always wonder if I'm doing a good mothering job, I know my baby is happy and the thought of having a second child is no longer frightening.*

Depression among men and women of all ages is thought to have various causes. The causes are sometimes referred to as psychological, behavioral, sociological, existential, and biological. Mental health experts define the theories like this:

- Psychological: This is depression that emerges as a result of negative thinking about oneself. It includes the loss of self-esteem, a feeling of helplessness, and lack of control in attaining one's goals.
- Behavioral: This is depression that results because a person has learned to act in a depressed manner, for example, a person who acts helpless and dependent on another.
- Sociological: Under this theory, a person becomes depressed because of the lack of a clear role in life or lack of control over life.

- Existential: Under this theory, depression results because of the loss of meaning and purpose in one's life.
- Biological: This depression is caused by an imbalance in chemicals in the brain that affect how we think and feel. This can be an inherited condition.

The causes of postpartum disorders are also thought to fall under these same various descriptions. For example, a biological cause might be hormonal fluctuations, including rapid change in estrogen and progesterone; and a sociological cause might describe a new mother who must place her infant in day care for long hours while she works in a job that holds no interest for her.

> *There seemed to be a physiological component to it. I had never taken antidepressants before and they worked so well for this depression. The cyclical nature of my depression also makes me wonder about the biological component. Talking didn't seem to help.*

Also, certain behaviors might cause the disorder. For example, you might have unrealistic expectations of parenting that have set you up for disappointment, coping problems, and depression.

> *I really thought that taking care of a baby would be as easy as the other challenges in my life. After all, I completed law school, passed the bar, and had done very well in my career. I was shocked that I felt so inept at parenting.*

Another psychological theory suggests that childbirth triggers the emergence of unresolved issues in a mother's life, such as her relationship with her mother or past sexual abuse.

> *My mother and I had never gotten along. I really felt like I didn't need her. I just went on with my life. But after I had my son, I really wished that I was closer*

*to her. It was hard to admit it, but I needed my
mother.*

And there are lifestyle causes of postpartum illness. The
depression could be a result of the difficult task of adjusting to a
new baby in addition to coping with other stressful circumstances,
such as a death in the family or financial or marital problems.

*I know I wouldn't have suffered postpartum depres-
sion had my husband not been mean to me during
my pregnancy, during labor, and during the first
three months after our daughter was born.*

HORMONES

Of all these explanations for postpartum illness, the theory that the
disorders are caused by hormone fluctuations has received the
greatest support. It also has caused the most controversy.

During the last week of pregnancy, a woman's metabolism
speeds up with increased amounts of estrogen and progesterone
circulating in the body. The pituitary gland, a pea-sized lobe
located at the base of the brain that is sometimes called the body's
master gland, must handle an increased blood supply and stimulate the production of hormones. But at birth, with the loss of the
placenta — the tissue that develops in the uterus during pregnancy
and helps nourish the growing fetus — the amounts of estrogen
and progesterone in the body fall off dramatically. The activity of
the pituitary subsides, also. The sudden drop in hormones and the
sluggishness of the pituitary gland could cause psychiatric symptoms such as anxiety or depression.

There is a great deal of conflicting evidence on how hormones
affect mood. Increasingly, studies show links between certain hormones and mood alterations. But if this is the cause of all postpartum illness, why does mood remain stable in many women after

childbirth? All women undergo substantial changes in hormones. Also, the hormonal theory does not explain the incidence of postpartum depression in fathers or in adoptive mothers, which has been reported in both groups following the arrival of a new baby.

Although studies connecting mood with hormone changes are inconclusive, anecdotal evidence supports this theory. For example, women who had suffered from a postpartum psychiatric illness were given estrogen or progesterone supplements in a subsequent pregnancy to curb the drastic drop in hormones. Studies show these prophylactic treatments have been largely successful in preventing depression or psychosis.[1]

Moreover, thyroid hormone imbalances are common after childbirth, and women with mood disturbances who have been treated with thyroid hormone supplements often recover quickly. Finally, one explanation for why some women have depression and others don't is that women may vary in their sensitivity to blood levels of various biochemical substances.

To further understand the biological cause of postpartum illness, doctors are now exploring the roles of menstruation, contraceptives, pregnancy, abortion, infertility, hysterectomy, and menopause and their links to depression over the lifecycle. With this kind of information, it may one day be possible to identify women who have a biological predisposition to postpartum illness before they even become pregnant.

"OUTSIDE" CAUSES

Experts seem to be more in agreement that outside factors — stress, society, and one's lifestyle — can contribute heavily to the cause of postpartum illness. The strongest factor associated with the development of the illness is the occurrence of recent stressful life events. And one shouldn't forget that, for most women, becoming a parent is a stressful life event.

The "normal" stress of parenthood is easily exacerbated. A new mother might be pushed over the edge by problems with her baby, spouse, parents, in-laws, boss, neighbors, friends, or even society in general. The cause of the illness can rarely be isolated to the mother alone and might lie in a complex web of relationships, lifestyle, and circumstances. Family interactions are sometimes a large part of the cause and must be addressed in treatment.

All these factors are important and can affect the severity of the illness and your own assessment of it. In fact, some experts suggest that a better term for postpartum depression would be *depression occurring in the postpartum period,* because that description would take into account the many, varied causes of the disorder.[2] It is possible that postpartum disorders are among the most sensitive of the biologically based mental disorders to environmental and lifestyle stress.

However, interactions of mind and body are not well understood, says Bernhard Pauliekhoff, a German physician. "The whole human being with body, soul, and mind must be studied if we are to achieve a suitable diagnosis and an optimal treatment." Postpartum illness, in particular, seems suited to a holistic view of mental health encompassing a variety of factors, including physiological, social, and cultural.

DIAGNOSING POSTPARTUM ILLNESS

Despite the lack of agreement on the causes of postpartum illness, the disorders can be treated successfully for almost all women. Perhaps the biggest problem is that too many doctors fail to recognize postpartum illness.

> *When I went for my six-week checkup after the birth of my son, I told the doctor that I was depressed, that I couldn't sleep and could barely take care of the baby. I told him I thought there was something*

wrong with me. He told me that it was normal to feel this way and that I should think about how lucky I am that I had a normal, healthy child. He told me I looked fine.

In an ideal world, a woman's obstetrician would notice a problem with her mood and would refer her to a psychiatrist or psychologist for treatment. The conversation might go something like this:

Obstetrician: "Hello, Janet! I can't believe it has been six weeks since Thomas was born. How is everything going?"

Janet: "Well, I'm awfully tired. But the baby is so sweet. I adore him."

Obstetrician: "Is he sleeping well?"

Janet: "Well, no. He's waking up a lot to nurse."

Obstetrician: "Do you get up for every feeding or does your husband help?"

Janet: "I'm breastfeeding, so I get up. Uh, my husband hasn't been that supportive. . . ."

Obstetrician: "I see. Things can be pretty tough during those first few weeks. Have you tried asking your husband to take one of the feedings? Perhaps you could use a breast pump and make up one bottle each night."

Janet: "He wouldn't do it . . . I . . . I really want to breastfeed . . . I'm so tired." Janet starts to cry.

Obstetrician: "I understand, Janet. I know we can find a way to deal with this."

There are many good doctors who offer their patients this kind of sensitivity, time, and resources. But what happens too often is that most women with postpartum disorders fall through the large crack between the specialties of obstetrics/gynecology and psychiatry.

"It's very much prevalent in postpartum illness that a woman will come and [the doctor] will see every single hazard and the clinician will still fall into the hole because he won't listen to what the woman is saying," says Dr. Deborah A. Sichel, a clinical instructor in psychiatry at Harvard Medical School and one of the nation's foremost experts on postpartum disorders. Moreover, many doctors adhere to old-fashioned myths about postpartum illness; for example, that only women who have medication at birth or only first-time mothers have it, or that having a cesarean section caused it. These are myths and have little to do with the development of most disorders.

Obstetricians may not see mental health matters as their responsibility. According to Robert Hickman, a marriage and family therapist and codirector of the Postpartum Mood Disorders Clinic in San Diego, "Obstetricians in general do not explore psycho-social issues during prenatal visits. The only thing that is expected, it seems, is the uncomplicated delivery of a normal infant who will enter a blissful postpartum period."

> *I had been in therapy for depression on and off since I was fifteen. Neither my psychiatrist or my obstetrician mentioned postpartum depression. My obstetrician and I never had any discussion about my psychological past. I never knew I was at high risk. No one ever asked me if I had had depression. I feel this illness was unnecessary.*

"Most obstetricians don't have great insight into the emotional problems of childbirth," notes Dr. David N. Danforth, a professor emeritus of ob-gyn at Northwestern University School of Medicine in Chicago. "Yet, the psychiatrists who do most of the writing about the problems don't have contact with the women themselves." Moreover, many psychiatrists also get inadequate training on mental disorders after childbirth. According to Sichel, some doctors simply downplay the seriousness of mood disorders after childbirth. "One of the biggest causes of women not getting well is that the syndrome is not recognized for being as serious as it is. Physicians will see this as being an adjustment disorder."

I kept going to doctors. I said, "Something is wrong. I can't stop crying." They all said, "Here, take these antidepressants and try to sleep." My periods affected my moods. I told the doctors, maybe it's hormones, and they looked at me like I was joking.

Other factors conspire to make diagnosis difficult. A woman may look nice and appear happy. She may claim all is well with her family. Even her symptoms of fatigue and insomnia might appear innocent because they are a common component of the postpartum period. "Sleeplessness and restlessness may be passed off as a by-product of excitement. . . . Confusion and headache may be blamed on loss of sleep," Hamilton says.

The mother may be given wrong advice: "Start exercising again. Get a babysitter and go away for the weekend." But if a physician's advice is inappropriate, symptoms could intensify and a woman may not get adequately diagnosed or treated.

Help is available for postpartum illness. But recovery begins when you and your family recognize you need help and find a caring health professional. More detailed information on treatment is offered in chapter seven. But to take that first step toward treatment, consider any of these recommendations:

- Discuss your problem with your obstetrician or midwife. He or she should be able to refer you to a psychologist or psychiatrist. If you "get the brush-off," try one of the other recommendations on this list.
- Call your baby's pediatrician and ask if he or she knows of a professional to refer you to for treatment of postpartum depression or anxiety.
- See the Resources section in the back of the book. Two organizations, Depression After Delivery and Postpartum Support International, are listed. These organizations should be able to refer you to an expert in your area. They can also put you in touch with other women in your area who have

experienced a postpartum illness. These women may be able to recommend a doctor.

- Call your city or county mental health office and inquire as to whether they can recommend an expert in postpartum depression.
- If you live near a university or teaching hospital, call the psychiatric departments of those institutions and inquire whether there is a postpartum expert on staff.

If you are already seeing a physician or therapist and that person or team is not meeting your needs, don't hesitate to find another doctor. Ask yourself these questions:

- Has the doctor given me and my family a treatment plan?
- Is he or she keeping me and my family informed of my progress?
- Has the doctor given me a complete physical, including laboratory tests? Has the doctor taken a full medical history, including my reproductive and mental health history and any history of addiction or abuse?
- Does the doctor or therapist seem knowledgeable about postpartum illness and seem comfortable discussing it?
- Can the doctor tell me something about past cases of postpartum illness he or she has treated?
- Does the doctor or therapist know of support groups for women with postpartum illness and their families?
- Is the doctor or therapist interested in my relationship with my baby and older children and in what my family is going through?
- Has my family been invited to participate in therapy?
- Has the doctor or therapist referred me to another specialist? (For example, a psychologist is not licensed to perform a physical examination and blood tests and should recommend that you at least see a physician to rule out any physical causes of your symptoms.)

YOU'RE NOT ALONE

It can be very hard to admit that all is not well. You may be embarrassed that you feel so sad or anxious during what is supposed to be such a joyful period of life. If you do talk about feelings, you might find others ignore them or feel uncomfortable with what you are saying. They might dismiss your concerns with the words: "It is normal to feel overwhelmed. You should be happy. You have a beautiful baby."

> *He was the ideal baby — perfect from day one. But I had sweating, shakiness, and fogginess. I couldn't cope with anything. I think I was more scared than anything. I thought I was losing my mind. And the doctors weren't any help at all.*

The possibility that your doctor will be unreceptive to your complaints or will downplay them may prevent you from raising the subject. The ability of depressed women to conceal their feelings is called "smiling depression," by English psychiatrist Joan Sneddon. These mothers try hard to dismiss their own feelings and think that if they carry on normally, they will eventually feel normal again.

> *My doctor, husband, and family urged me to talk with a professional, but it was so difficult to accept the fact that I desperately needed help. I had a background in social work and spent many years trying to help others. I was ashamed that something bigger than myself had encompassed my being and I had no control over it.*

If you compare yourself with other mothers who appear fine, you may feel even more embarrassed about your own needs. Writing about her own postpartum depression, Dr. Katharina Dalton, an expert on mood disorders and the reproductive cycle, says: "I know how lonely I felt, surrounded by all the other happy, competent new mothers who clearly had not the slightest difficulty managing their homes, their work, their new babies, or themselves."

When the mother is silent, it may fall to the husband and family to help her. Families should remember that depressed mothers often exhibit clues that they are suffering. "The most common sign of their depression is complaining of their worthlessness as mothers," says Jane Price, author of *Motherhood: What It Does To Your Mind.* "These complaints tend to be accepted at face value rather than compared with reality and questioned, hence the mother's sadness escapes without comment. Many women report a state of 'feeling nothing' for themselves, their babies or for anyone or anything."

You may not realize you are depressed because parenthood represents such a profound change in your life. New mothers typically believe that they should be happy and have no place to categorize or process the more negative reactions to motherhood. "[Women] believe that they are just leading a lower quality of life bogged down by utter exhaustion and irritability — a sadly changed character. It is all too easy to blame their condition on the extra work that the baby brings into their new life," Dalton says.

Given the blessing of a new baby, you may feel you have no reason to feel sad or tense. "There is little in her temperature chart or in objective findings to justify this discomfort," Hamilton says. "Her physicians, her relatives, and her own common sense tell her that she has no reason to be ill. Nevertheless, she feels sick."

I felt really bad because he was the perfect baby. I felt I had no reason to feel like I did. He slept through the night. I was the one who didn't sleep through the night.

Because there has been so little public discussion of postpartum illness, it's not unusual for a woman to think she is completely alone in her misery. "Each woman with postnatal depression believes that it is only she who can't keep the house in order, has sleepless nights, shouts at her children and nags incessantly at her partner," says Dr. Deborah Sharp, a London-based physician. Although all mothers feel this way from time to time, it is the frequency and intensity of these feelings that distinguishes healthy women from women who are ill.

OVERCOMING THE STIGMA

There are two responses I get when I tell people what happened to me. One is, "Oh. Mental Illness. Back Off." The other is, "You know, I think that happened to me. What are your symptoms? I never got any help."

Since you probably have never had a mental disorder, the idea of seeking mental health counseling or treatment may seem frightening. And if you have always viewed yourself as competent and independent, it may be hard to ask for help. Try to resist the thought that therapy is for helpless individuals. Getting treatment for this disorder is no different than seeking help for high blood pressure or painful menstrual cycles.

It is crucial to identify and treat the disorder early, since the longer the illness goes on, the more difficult recovery might be. What's more, the consequences of ignoring your mental and emotional well-being can be profound. The longer the illness is left untreated, the greater the risk of long-term repercussions to you, your baby, and the bonds that link your family together.

Things sure get out of whack fast when there's a new baby crying all night long.

There are signs that the medical profession is waking up to the importance of this health problem. More researchers are pursuing the questions surrounding postpartum disorders. And many women are demanding answers and getting the help they need.

Members of support groups for postpartum patients and their families, and interested professionals — such as Depression After Delivery (Morrisville, Pennsylvania) and Postpartum Support International (Santa Barbara, California) — have done much to alert the public to the disorder by giving candid television and newspaper interviews. (Addresses and telephone numbers for support organizations are listed in the Resources section at the back of this book.)

You can and will find help. But as a society, we still have a long way to go in understanding the biological underpinnings of postpartum depression and in learning how to treat new mothers with the care they need and deserve.

CHAPTER THREE

Adjusting to Motherhood

She had always wanted children.

To Maria, the image of a house, a husband, and a family was the ultimate dream in life. After thirty-two years, she had developed a respectable career as a saleswoman. She had met the right man and married. And now, she was having a baby.

"I thought, 'I finally have everything I want.' When we found out I was pregnant, we went out to eat and celebrated, then came home and called everyone we knew to tell them the news. We couldn't keep it a secret!"

Maria had expected her pregnancy would be a glorious time. She envisioned shopping leisurely for cute maternity clothes and wasn't worried about what the growing baby inside her would do to her trim figure. But in her fifth month of pregnancy, Maria began to bleed and doctors diagnosed a condition called placenta previa. She was ordered to remain home and in bed until her delivery date.

"That was the last thing I expected," says Maria, a soft-spoken woman with large brown eyes. "Having to leave my job four months earlier than I had planned really hurt us financially. And I never

got to do all the things I had looked forward to doing: wallpapering the nursery, shopping for baby clothes and furniture. I didn't even have a chance to talk to other people about the baby and share my anticipation. I didn't get to wear half of the nice maternity clothes I had bought for work."

Maria's due date finally arrived and she underwent a scheduled cesarean section. A son, Joseph, was born to Maria and her husband, Manny. The couple rejoiced at their healthy little boy.

Maria expected to be sore and exhausted from her surgery. And this time, her expectations were right on target. She was unable to breastfeed her child until the third day. And on her fourth day of hospitalization she was discharged — her insurance carrier would pay for only four days of hospitalization unless Maria had complications. In fact, Maria had recovered well from childbirth. But, as a nurse wheeled her down the hall from the shiny, new hospital, Maria felt tired, tearful, and overwhelmed.

The day was hot and humid and Manny and Maria struggled to strap the car seat into their car while the nurse held the baby, trying to shield him from the sun. The couple began to argue about which way the seat should be buckled in. Finally, after what seemed to be a major hassle, the new family was on its way home. But they were a fragile unit. Everything, it seemed to Maria, was turning into a major hassle.

"When we got home, I immediately went into the bedroom, got into bed, and tried to breastfeed the baby. Feeding had been going pretty well in the hospital. But now that we were home, I was really struggling. My breasts had become engorged, and

feeding was excruciatingly painful. That on top of being so sore from my surgery! I cried most of that first day home."

Meanwhile, Manny stood by, feeling somewhat helpless and looking for something to do. He had arranged to take a week's vacation from work. But with Maria breastfeeding his son, he felt shut out and somewhat unimportant. Maria seemed to reject whatever advice or suggestions he offered. Neither parent had envisioned that the first few days home with a new baby could be so tiring and tense.

Maria felt that her house had been turned upside down. Expecting to love and mother and confidently care for her baby, she felt she was being controlled by this 8-pound being. In the days after her return home, she had let her own self-care go while frantically trying to feed and calm her baby. Now she still felt sore, tired, unattractive, and overburdened with housework. The baby's laundry seemed to grow by itself. She seemed to be running the washing machine all day long. Each day, she set aside the morning newspaper, hoping to read it but never getting the chance. She felt anxious to write and mail her birth announcements, fill in the baby book, and send thank-you cards for the gifts and flowers the family had received. But when she looked at the pile of notes and packages and newspapers on her dining room table, she felt she would never regain control of her life.

"At work, I usually felt challenged and happy when I knew I had to work hard that day, completing orders, making phone calls, and planning my schedule. But at home, I couldn't seem to complete one single task. At first I tried to make lists of things

I needed to do. But that only made me feel I was falling further behind."

To Manny, Maria seemed like a different person. She never smiled, except at the baby. And he felt like a failure. Seeing her husband's look of sadness and bewilderment only added to Maria's guilt. She couldn't make anyone happy! She began to doubt her decision to have a baby so soon after the couple had married. Maybe she wasn't even cut out to be a parent, she thought to herself many times.

By the time Joseph was four weeks old, however, Maria no longer felt that she was going to burst into tears at any moment. Slowly, almost imperceptibly, Joseph had settled into a predictable and easy feeding schedule.

"I don't know if there was a turning point when I began to feel like myself again. But I do think that getting the breastfeeding down finally gave me some more self-confidence. Before that, I felt like I was the worst mother in the world! And, as the baby fed better, he slept better. And I began to get more sleep. Sleep helped more than anything. As soon as I started getting close to seven hours of sleep a night, I quit crying at the drop of a hat."

Feeling that she was beginning to control her life again, Maria began to call friends and make plans. Manny breathed a sigh of relief, too, and began to enjoy his son.

The maternity blues lasted about three weeks for Maria, although she felt that her adjustment to motherhood had only just begun. She realized that parenthood would always be filled with ups and downs.

"When people ask me about the baby now, I tell the truth: It had been hard at first but things were *getting better. The first month was a disaster. Manny and I had no idea it would be this hard, this unpredictable. If I learned anything about being a mother, it's that you can't make rigid plans. You have to be laid back. Unfortunately, I'm kind of a hyper person. But I think becoming a mother has taught me to be more patient."*

Your adjustment to motherhood can be an important contributing factor in postpartum depression — whether or not hormones play a role. The stresses, strain, and exhaustion might be the final straw for a woman already vulnerable to depression. Even for some healthy women without a biological vulnerability to depression, the task of becoming a mother can lead to serious introspection, and sometimes, a cascade of negative emotions.

While many mental health experts believe that hormones play at least some role in some postpartum disorders, they do not downplay the importance of understanding what a new mother must cope with in the first weeks and months following childbirth. The first year of motherhood isn't always what women anticipate. In a survey of almost five hundred mothers of one-year-olds, 25 percent described the transition as difficult. And most of the women rated their relationships with their spouses and friends, their physical and financial well-being, their desire to work outside the home, their feelings of competence as a mother, and the degree of help they were getting from their husbands as significantly lower after one year of parenthood. The researchers attributed this slip in satisfaction to inflated expectations about parenthood. And, the more a woman expected, the more likely she was to end up depressed with her life.[1]

COPING WITH THE UNEXPECTED

Many mothers experience some degree of sadness and anxiety after childbirth because of the fantasies they have constructed around this event. Before you had your baby you probably rarely heard about the stress, the hardships, and the draining aspects of parenting an infant — other than the cheerful warnings that "your life will change" or "you won't get any sleep." Usually, only the positive aspects of motherhood — and there are many — are discussed. But to deny that it is sometimes difficult to be a mother is to be left unprepared and vulnerable to disappointment.

> *I had a difficult labor. I had a lot of back pain. But I had made a meditation tape with my own voice on it, and that helped a lot. When my daughter was born it was the most beautiful, emotional experience that I've ever had. As soon as she came out, my husband and I started crying. I couldn't believe this beautiful girl came out of me. But I had no idea how hard those first few months would be. When we left the hospital, my daughter was crying and my husband and I were bickering over how to comfort her. I felt inadequate and inept. The baby was a horrible sleeper. She would wake up every two to three hours. I was exhausted — a zombie. After I breastfed her I would have to lie down. I didn't have any energy. I couldn't even drive. I couldn't stand hearing her cry in the car. I never even took her to the grocery store because if she cried I felt I couldn't stand it. The isolation became phenomenal. I felt buried under the laundry, the meals . . . We thought we were so prepared for this baby. But I had a lot more confidence during my pregnancy than after it.*

"Traditionally, women have been misled by a too-rosy picture of motherhood and, as a result, they have been left unprepared for the widely experienced difficulties," say Lyn DelliQuadri and Kati Breckenridge in their book *The New Mother Care*, which focuses on some myths of motherhood. Indeed, the first reaction of the new mother, appalled that her experience is so contrary to her expectations, is this: "Why didn't they tell me it was like this?"

We were thirty-seven when we got married and thirty-nine when we had the baby. After I had the baby, I was afraid to admit my real feelings. If you didn't have these high expectations maybe you wouldn't get so depressed . . . I thought my husband would do more. He did less. I resented that I had no time for myself.

More enlightened mental health professionals and physicians call the birth of a child only slightly less stressful than the sudden death of a loved one. It is this view that must be accepted if women are to learn to ask for and obtain all the support and resources necessary to make a smoother transition to motherhood.

Glorious expectations of motherhood can collide with reality from the moment of conception on. Like many women, you might have been physically ill during pregnancy with nausea, fatigue, swelling, backache, and a number of other ills. The birth experience may not have gone the way you expected. The natural childbirth movement, which swept the country in the 1960s and 1970s, brought many good changes to birthing. Women now have so much more control and choices in childbirth. But the movement may have innocently led some women to believe that childbirth can take any form they choose — that it can always be pain and drug free, and they won't need stitches or much medical intervention. This belief sets an impossibly high standard that few women can hope to achieve. Many women are left feeling depressed and that they have failed when they cannot live up to this ideal.

You may also have found you were unprepared for your reaction to your child. The feelings of intense love and joy that you expected to have may have escaped you as you looked at this child who was a far cry from the version in your dreams. Once at home with the new baby, the fatigue is often greater than most women have ever experienced or could imagine. The baby's first sweet smile may be eight weeks away, and you may not have been fore-warned that a new baby would make great demands on you when you were at your lowest, both physically and emotionally. Your dis-couragement during this period is entirely natural!

Nowadays, new mothers often leave the hospital in one day if they have had a vaginal birth and in two or three days if they have had a cesarean section. In some areas of the United States, health insurers have requested that mothers and infants be discharged after twelve hours for a normal vaginal birth — making birth a mere pit stop. Many states have enacted laws to thwart this trend.

Think of how our society's attitudes about childbirth have changed. In 1970, new mothers were allowed four days of rest and recuperation following a vaginal birth (almost eight days for a cesarean section). The current trend of tossing mother and baby from the hospital has gone so far that many health organizations, including the American College of Obstetricians and Gynecolo-gists, have protested it. This trend has been fostered by heightened concern about health care costs. But it also reflects the view that childbirth is a natural event and that a pregnant or birthing mother is not an invalid. Though this is true, it seems the pendulum has swung too far. Even if you have arranged for help at home, the sheer physical demands of pregnancy and childbirth and caring for an infant may wear down much of your energy, spirit, and enthusiasm. And yet few people stop to consider what effect this physical and emotional stress might have on your mind, mood, and perceptions.

Women report that they cope with many side effects of child-birth long after they leave the hospital, including fatigue, hemor-rhoids, constipation, sweating, dizziness, hot flashes, and acne. Several of these disorders — particularly dizziness, fatigue, and digestive problems — frequently persist beyond one month. Moreover, some symptoms of childbirth emerge weeks after the birth. These can include hair loss, sexual dysfunction, and respira-tory problems. One study of almost one hundred women found that 25 percent felt they had not physically recovered from child-birth six months after delivery.[2]

The baby sleeps only thirty minutes a day. I like to take a shower every day. But it has to be every third day because of the baby. It kills me. And she's into everything. I have to ignore my six-year-old. It's all so stressful.

It's impossible to separate mind and body. If your muscles are tense, you may become more tense. If you don't eat nourishing food, you may become tired more easily. If your body is sluggish and inactive, it may have a depressing effect on your thoughts.

For many weeks, the infant will give little back in the way of a response. But remember that the smiles and coos of a three-month-old baby will hearten you, and a full night's sleep will help curb the fatigue. There is much you can do to combat the feeling of being overwhelmed and stressed out. Here are some suggestions:

- Accept help when it's offered. Tell the individual offering help what it is you need the most (for example, "Could you take Shelly to preschool this week?" or "When you go to the grocery store today, could you pick up a few things for me?"
- Likewise, if you have help in your home (a mother or a mother-in-law perhaps), be clear and firm about how you can best be assisted. This can be a touchy area — you don't want to offend someone who is trying to help. Try saying, for example, "Donna, you're such a big help. What I really need for you to do now is fold that laundry while I feed Ashley." If a conflict remains, ask your spouse to intervene. Your husband should be a buffer to keep unnecessary stresses from you in these first few weeks after childbirth.
- Make your needs known — to yourself, your spouse, and others. Bottling up feelings of frustration will only make the days ahead harder. Tell your husband, "Everything seems so chaotic right now. It would give me some peace of mind if you could keep the house straightened up."
- If you don't have help, get it. This is not a good time to fret over balancing your monthly household budget. Babysitters

and take-out meals may never seem more valuable to you and your spouse as they will during this period.

- If you're having trouble with the baby, such as feeding problems or colic, call your pediatrician often and be assertive in requesting advice. You will probably never need your pediatrician more than during the first six months of your baby's life. You won't wear out your welcome!

- Do try to rest whenever you can. New mothers are often "revved up" — after all, it's so exciting to have a new baby. But fatigue will accumulate. If you can't nap, at least lie down occasionally. Remember even a twenty-minute nap can help you feel better.

- Eat good food. Avoid too much sugar, caffeine, or alcohol. Eat whole grains, fruit, and vegetables. Make eating a priority. Yes, you are very busy. But you need sustenance. Don't diet now. The first eight weeks of the postpartum period is really a poor time to be concerned about your weight. You don't need that pressure right now. TV hostess Mary Hart returned to her job on *Entertainment Tonight* interviewing movie stars in front of millions of people two months after having her baby. She was unconcerned that she had not lost all her pregnancy weight, confidently saying that she intended to ease back to her normal weight. What a great endorsement for the normalcy of weight gain surrounding pregnancy!

- Find someone to talk to about your feelings and what you're experiencing. A sympathetic listener is invaluable. Be honest about your feelings; confront them. If you feel touchy, say so. But try also to think about the positive things that happened to you today.

- You may be tired, but try to exercise. The exercise can consist of just going out for a walk or a stroll with your baby. Many mothers who have experienced postpartum illness have remarked that walks in the fresh air are very therapeutic. And research suggests that the effects of exercise on your brain can actually mitigate depression. If you can, leave the baby with someone and go by yourself.

With the trend in shorter maternity stays in the hospital and home births, a new industry has sprung up to meet the needs of the new mother and her family. These parent-care services are available in most cities and are sometimes called Motherlove or Mother-Care Services. Trained women, often mothers themselves, provide such services as tending to the new mother's medical needs, helping with the baby, answering questions, making sure the mother rests, providing breastfeeding instruction, and preparing some meals. The services generally cost from $10 to $30 per hour. To find a service near you, contact the National Association of Postpartum Care Services, a clearinghouse for eighty programs. (See the Resources section in the back of the book for the address.)

THE MYTHICAL MOTHER

What should a mother be like? What image do you conjure up? You may think of your own mother. But your image may also be gleaned from advertising, movies, television, childhood stories, and fairy tales. A little girl playing with a doll is dreaming up her vision of the perfect mother. She will have many years to embellish the image, constructing this picture in her mind right up through her pregnancy.

Sometimes we need to dispel our lofty images in order to accept and enjoy the true nature of motherhood. DelliQuadri and Breckenridge describe three myths linked to motherhood: maternal instinct, motherlove, and maternal fulfillment.

Maternal instinct is described as a biological drive to have children, love the children unconditionally, and know intrinsically how to care for them. Motherlove describes the self-sacrifice, untiring service, and undying patience that spouts endlessly from a mother. Maternal fulfillment is the "undefinable sense of satisfaction that can be acquired only with a baby." The baby becomes the source of gratification and fulfillment, and the single experience a woman needs to be happy and complete.

These mythical attributes of motherhood were created by society in ages past to promote and facilitate the birth of more children who could contribute to the family economy. They remain tightly woven into the fabric of modern society. And yet the idea that mothering comes naturally and is carried out with little sweat or strain is a real disservice to women. The problem is that if you believe in these myths, you may expect mothering to be easy. And it rarely is. If you expect mothering to be easy and find it isn't, you may blame yourself and consider yourself a failure.

"The mythology holds that mothering is 'intuitive' and 'natural.' A mother is expected to respond intuitively to the baby's needs so that the baby is happy and contented and does not cry," say members of the Pacific Post Partum Support Society in Vancouver.

I read the books [on childrearing]. One says one thing and one says another. She's waking up every hour all night long. I have lost my confidence. I have lost my common sense. Who said that this motherhood thing is a natural instinct? I don't have it. I don't know what to do.

Many experts refer to the postpartum period as a "crisis." For some women, the crisis consists of realizing that what worked in their lives before no longer works.

I had had this wonderful career for sixteen years, but after the birth of my son, my whole life seemed to turn upside down. For a long time after he was born, I struggled with feelings of ambivalence about having had the baby. At times I thought, "Why did I ever think I could do this?" After a few months at home taking care of the baby, I began looking for ways to feel in control of my life again, looking for ways to structure my life. I started feeling better after about six months. By that time I had "mommy" friends. I made dinner dates with mom-

*mies and their kids. I gave myself permission to
talk mommy talk. My marriage changed, too. I feel
like after having my son I finally grew up. We were
twenty-two when we got married. It's been an
adjustment as far as our marriage. We have had to
make sure we had the time for heart-to-heart talks
to express the loss of our freedom. Our marriage is
definitely different.*

Ironically, the woman who is expected to make the most
trouble-free transition to motherhood is the one who may be most
at risk for postpartum depression. A woman with a very controlling personality who plans her pregnancy, attends prenatal classes
with her husband, and has the support of her husband at childbirth may be the one most set up for disappointment. She expects
disappointment the least and may be shocked that she cannot control motherhood the way she could control her life before the baby.

Sometimes this realization that being a mom is not so easy is
accompanied by anger. Anger at yourself, your husband, and your
baby is one of the most disconcerting, and yet common, emotions
of motherhood.

*I started feeling rage. I got so frustrated with my
older son's behavior. I got physically out of control
with him. I'd become so angry I'd grab and squeeze
his arm. I wanted to pick him up and throw him. I
felt so guilty shaking him. I thought, boy, I am really
out of control.*

You and your baby may not necessarily be a perfect fit at first.
The mother and baby relationship demands compromise. Neither
will be perfect. But if you're not prepared to work out a compromise with your fantasy of motherhood, negative emotions become
the response to this uncomfortable fit.

"Not only are women self-critical of their negative emotional response to motherhood, they also quickly discover that

everyone else is highly critical of it too," says Jane Price, author of the book *Motherhood: What It Does to Your Mind.* "This leads many women to cover up their feelings, to think of their feelings as bad or shameful and to deny them, to themselves as well as to others. Buried feelings do not go away, they lurk under the surface looking for some other way out. Some women are lucky enough to have friends, hobbies or work as 'vents' for the black side of mothering but those women who have no safety valves have an increasing build-up of pressure in their psyches. Many women have said to me, 'I just want to open my mouth and scream and scream to let all the bad feelings out.'"

> *I couldn't understand why I was feeling so depressed and so resentful of the baby. I felt horrible about myself. I kept asking myself, "What is wrong with me? Why am I feeling this way toward this beautiful little girl I had wanted all my life?" I didn't tell anyone how I felt. I was very ashamed. My pediatrician noticed something was really wrong with me. He said, "What is wrong with you?" I said I didn't know. I was afraid he'd take her from me. But I started crying in his office. The pediatrician referred me to a psychologist. I told the psychologist that I should be locked away. I was ashamed of how I was feeling. A good mother doesn't feel that way . . . If I had learned that the postpartum depression wasn't my fault, maybe I would have been able to discuss my symptoms sooner. But I was embarrassed. I felt it was my fault.*

Try not to judge yourself against your expectations of motherhood. The postpartum depression that ensues when reality collides with fantasy is not unique to mothers who give birth. If you're an adoptive mother you too may have to dismantle all the myths and fantasies surrounding motherhood in order to accept yourself as you are and credit yourself for the many things you do well.

When you're tired, frustrated, or overwhelmed, give yourself some positive messages:

- Remember that you need not live up to any image or ideal of motherhood. You will be a good enough mother just the way you are.
- Remind yourself that you're doing the best you can.
- Throw away your lists. Stop checking off your accomplishments and "failures." If you get one thing done today that you wanted to accomplish, applaud. You've had a good day.
- Don't beat yourself up because you snapped at your husband or lost your patience with your three-year-old. Apologize and forget about it.
- Do something nice for yourself. Get a babysitter and go out to dinner. Don't feel guilty about leaving your infant with a sitter!
- Don't feel it's incumbent on you to do everything. Others have responsibilities, too. Remind them if they forget.
- Lower your standards. Ask yourself if it really matters if the house isn't dusted this week or that your children haven't had a green vegetable in three days.
- Don't worry about your physical appearance unless it makes you feel better to dress up.

Remember that parenting — in this society — is something you learn on the job. It takes time. Mistakes are involved. There is no such thing as perfect. Mothers today are less prepared for mothering than their own mothers — even less prepared than women in preindustrialized societies. It's not your fault. It's just the way our society is, and it's something we, as a society, need to address.

One way to prepare yourself for what lies ahead is to talk to other mothers. You will benefit tremendously by being allowed to release your thoughts and by hearing that many new mothers feel as you do.

Sometimes it's hard to talk to your friends because, on the surface, they appear so happy and competent and you may feel disorganized and lost. But, if you break the ice, you'll often find your friends share similar experiences. We live in a culture that does not encourage close female contact. Indeed, instead of supporting each other, women who work outside the home and women who remain at home to care for children full-time frequently wage a war of words in the media over which group is happier, more fulfilled, and has the most well-adjusted children. How horribly self-defeating to all. Instead, it should be pointed out that even the most untrained parents raise fine children in spite of the lack of preparation for parenthood and the lack of support from society.

Candid, honest discussion about parenting would help in other ways, too. Experts suggest that until parents learn to speak openly about their experiences and feelings, there is little more that can be learned about raising children to be well adjusted and healthy. Understanding the realities of motherhood would help society identify what needs to be done to nurture the entire family unit. To understand, accept, and prepare for the downside is to be able to more clearly experience and cherish the many joys of mothering.

Who Am I Now?

Sandy was thirty-six and a psychotherapist with a booming practice in an affluent suburb. She and her businessman husband had been married fourteen years. For almost four years, they had discussed having a child. After experiencing difficulties conceiving, the couple was thrilled to learn a baby girl was on the way. They took childbirth preparation classes and rejoiced when the healthy infant was born.

Sandy took only two days off after the birth and then began seeing a client or two each day at the office in her home. But the demands of her baby and her job began to wear her down. She was exhausted, cried easily, and wondered what had become of the pulled-together professional who helped other people solve their problems. She felt her husband wasn't helping her enough and was dismayed when her babysitter quit. She felt she had no one to turn to for help. "It was so strange for me switching roles, being the career woman for so long, out there being a teacher, a facilitator, a counselor. It was a switch to be so needy. I felt the need to be mothered. I remember when my daughter was three months old going to a Gymboree class. I remember sitting in the circle and talking to myself and saying 'Sandy, it's okay to sit here and just be a member. You don't have to lead.' I didn't want other moms to know I felt so awful."

You may sometimes feel like you're not the same person since the birth of your baby. It's not just that the additional title of "mother" has been added to your personal resume. Something else has happened. You may have found strengths you never knew you had and weaknesses that you abhor. You may feel differently about your job, coworkers, husband, best friend, and your mother.

When you become a mother you deal with a change in identity, increased responsibility, decreased autonomy, a change in the marital relationship, a new relationship with an infant, and a change in career or the need to reconcile the loss of your career. Some women cope well with these changes and others have difficulty. Experts have identified some character traits that might make the transition harder:

- being overcontrolling
- having an obsessive personality

- having prior unresolved developmental issues
- harboring unresolved grief
- having a history of prior difficulty adapting to a crisis
- having a conflictual relationship with your mother
- having difficulties identifying with your mother
- having conflicts regarding femininity and motherhood
- being a single parent

You may become overwhelmed and disconcerted with this new and unfamiliar picture of yourself as a mother. Part of this new "you" involves adapting to a very different schedule. The time schedule of mothering may be unlike anything you have experienced before. There is no schedule. You may have a feeling of having accomplished nothing at the end of the day. The repetition of tasks and the never-ending supply of jobs to be done can be overwhelming if you're the kind of person who once neatly scratched off each completed task in your leather-bound organizer. Caring for babies is emotional and changeable, and has no set procedure. Many women are not used to this type of role. You're not the first!

> *I became more obsessed with having to know every-*
> *thing that was going on. I wanted things in control.*

Some experts suggest that becoming a new mother is an identity crises similar to that of retirement.

> *It's a dramatic change from having a career to*
> *becoming a mom. It's a change from having control*
> *over every degree of my life to having very little con-*
> *trol over any aspect of my life. And even if you get a*
> *raise once a year at work, that's more recognition*
> *than you get as a mom.*

A big part of the problem with this new identity is that it is thrust on you so suddenly. You may have envisioned your maternity leave as relaxing and enjoyable, allowing you some time to thoughtfully adjust and re-evaluate your life. But the demands of the first few months leave little time for introspection and casual adjustment. Some women feel they are spinning out of control. When they look in the mirror and see the haggard face and spit-up stained T-shirt, many will indeed wonder what has become of their former selves.

Some women expect motherhood to transform them into something better than their past selves. Although becoming a mother offers the opportunity to achieve tremendous growth and profound fulfillment, the birth of a child will not in and of itself bestow fulfillment and satisfaction on a woman. Motherhood won't solve pre-existing problems of insecurity over who you are. One study, in fact, found poor self-esteem to be a powerful factor in the development of postpartum depression.[3]

THE CHANGING MARRIAGE

> *I don't think either my husband or I knew how to*
> *co-parent. He didn't know what to do, and I didn't*
> *know how to ask him. I felt, well, I'm at home, I*
> *should be able to handle it.*

In some families, fathers are just not expected to help much or alter their lifestyles after having a baby. This points out a true tragedy and weakness in the American family portrait, because research continually suggests that the contributions of the father to the family, if he is present, are critical to the health of the family. In the weeks and months after childbirth, a father's contributions include becoming a "barrier" between the mother and baby and the outside world — that "world" being financial strains and people who can cause the mother stress and disrupt her time with the baby.

Many women are upset with the response of their partners to parenthood and their increasing needs, feeling their husbands are not supportive, empathic, or helpful enough. Inadequate support and a distance from one's husband are important factors in the development of postpartum illness.

It is a great strength in a marriage to be flexible and respond to each other's changing needs. The husband or partner needs to nurture the new mother and develop a relationship with his child. If a husband can nurture a baby successfully, this frees the mother to begin a stage in which she can separate from the baby, after the intense period of bonding in infancy, to resume her work, relationships with others, and interests.

Many fathers need some direction. They, too, have not been trained for becoming parents. Their own fathers probably weren't great role models for being an involved parent. Men may feel awkward and useless. Couples need to talk about what the father can do to help. He should be made to feel as important as he is. He needs goals and clear ideas of your expectations.

> *We were married ten years before we had her. I guess I thought that things would be sort of the same but that she comes with us in a backpack. It's not like that at all.*

Instead of the baby linking you and your husband closer, which many couples believe will happen, the chaos and strain may make you feel like strangers. If you're at home all day with a baby, you may also feel lonely and confined.

> *My husband was too busy to help me but still expected good meals and a clean house. I felt overwhelmed by all the things I had to do just to care for the baby. Soon I realized that my husband and I weren't even talking to each other anymore.*

Marriage adjustments after having a baby are to be expected. Expect some rough days. The key to keeping your conflicts to a minimum, however, is talking. Of course, who has the time to talk? Make communication a priority. Try to identify a time of day when things seem the calmest — breakfast time is often good — and give each other attention — discuss your thoughts and feelings and solutions to your problems. Remember that humor is a very useful tool. One woman who gave birth to twins was given this sage advice by her obstetrician:

1. Hire help in the home, and don't be cheap.
2. Get away alone with your husband frequently, even if it's just an overnight trip.
3. Establish a house rule that only one of you at a time can be in a bad mood.

REMEMBERING YOUR MOTHER

The baby is me. And I am my mom.

Next to your husband, the person you may need the most during the postpartum period is your own mother. While you take care of your demanding new infant — a task that can consume the majority of your day and night — who takes care of you? Who makes sure that you are eating well? Who answers the telephone so you can take a nap while the baby is napping? Who reassures you that all babies cry and that you will certainly be a wonderful mother? Your own mother might best fill that role.

Many women, however, do not have the support of their mothers in the postpartum period. For some, it is because their mothers live far away and simply cannot be with them. Others have lost their mothers. But some do not have the kind of relationship with their mothers that allows them to accept or receive whatever warmth, love, and support a mother can give.

Moreover, childbirth can also stir up long dormant feelings you have about your own mother. Did you feel loved and cared for as a child? Did you mimic your mother? Is your mother a role model? Or is your mother an example of what you do not want to become? Some women don't want to be like their mothers and fear childbirth will cause them to become their mothers. Your opinion of your own mother influences how you will perceive yourself as a mother. You will remember aspects of how you were parented, store these memories away, and recall them when you become a parent. Your basic assumptions and expectations of mothering arise out of this experience and memory.

> *I feel like I've been suffering from depression since I was five years old. I remember when I was five my mother would become frustrated and angry with me and ask, "Why are you such a sullen child?" I knew I was unhappy but I didn't know why. I had such poor self-esteem when I was growing up. I didn't feel loved or important. My parents were alcoholics and there was a lot of emotional abuse at home. My father was physically abusive. My mother was emotionally abusive. I wasn't able to find myself. I met my husband when we were sixteen. I was twenty-one when we got married. I didn't know who I was when I had my child. That's why I had a baby. I thought it would give me some iden-tity. We were twenty-two when we had the baby. My husband's childhood was pretty bad, too. Neither of us had good role models for marriage or parent-hood. We've had to learn how to become parents. What our parents did with us was very screwed up.*

"Whether we are male or female, parents or childless, the care of children reawakens our buried selves," says Jane Swigart, author of *The Myth of the Bad Mother.* "For better or worse, child care pulls us in two directions: outward toward the children we tend and inward toward our own earliest experiences of being cared for. Our first, most intense relationship with our mother often remains unconscious and inaccessible until we have children, at which point all the longings and ambivalence we felt toward her rise up in us again."

If you had insufficient mothering as a child or your mother has died, the postpartum period can represent a painful time. Or you may instead re-evaluate your relationship with your mother as you begin to form a new picture of your childhood. Giving birth may help you understand the pressures and feelings experienced by your mother. You may see your mother in a new, softer light when you become a mother. You may have the urge to reconcile with your mother in order to become comfortable and capable as a mother yourself. "The presence of a baby often provides a new battleground for mother-daughter conflicts as well as a resurgence of feelings of anger, rejection, deprivation, or rivalry. These are expressions of the need for reconciliation, a need that is bound to find a way to make itself known," DelliQuadri and Breckenridge say.

MOTHERS AND RELATIONSHIPS

Why are relationships with her husband and mother so extremely crucial, so sensitive, to a new mother? According to a fascinating new theory developed over the past two decades by a group of feminist psychologists, a woman's spirit, her psyche, her sense of self-worth, is dependent on the success of her relationship with others.

To arrive at this conclusion, this group of theorists first asked themselves whether a woman's psychological development is different from a man's. They believe the basic problem in understanding healthy psychological development in women is that current developmental theory is written by men, for men. Although this theory is debated, psychologists suggest that a women's sense of self becomes very much organized around being able to make and then to maintain relationships.

The pioneering work in 1976 by Jean Baker Miller, a clinical professor of psychiatry at Boston University of Medicine, titled

Toward a New Psychology of Women, is based on a theme called the self-in-relation theory. This is a rather stilted name for the idea that a woman's self-esteem is organized around and developed based on her relationships with other people.

The belief is that from early in her upbringing, a female child's sense of self reflects what is happening between her and other people. While growing up, she is encouraged to empathize with others. Maintaining relationships becomes the most important thing to her. And self-esteem and self-worth are closely tied to the development of relationships.

Women with successful relationships find a pathway to healthy psychological development; and those with unsuccessful relationships may blame themselves, feel like failures, and exhaust themselves in their efforts to have perfect relationships, thus suffering from a range of negative mental health effects — including a high degree of depression.

A woman may become depressed when she does not experience growth and satisfaction from the effort she puts into her relationships. Although relationships bring women great satisfaction and happiness, relationship strains constitute a greater risk factor for depression. "Women are expected to respond to the pain and the needs of others, whether or not their own needs for support and validation are met," says Janet L. Surrey, director of psychiatry at McLean Hospital in Belmont, Massachusetts. A woman so wrapped up in the concerns of others, so eager to meet the expectations of other people, will not listen to her own wishes and needs and will not even really know herself.

What we can learn from the self-in-relation theory is that some depression can result from a new mother's attempt to live up to what is expected of her in today's society. New mothers don't become depressed because of their babies. Their unhappiness stems more from living in a world in which, they soon realize, they will receive little help or support. How society treats new mothers is very important to their emotional well-being, as we shall see in the next chapter.

CHAPTER FOUR

Society and Motherhood

In Guatemala, you're not supposed to do anything for the first forty days after childbirth. For the next three months, you're only supposed to do things gradually. Here in America, when you have a baby, if you're not back up in three days people ask, "What's wrong with you?"

Much has changed for families in the last thirty years. The lives of new mothers today are a far cry from those of our mothers. In the 1950s and '60s, many women had several children and often did not attempt to work outside the home. In most neighborhoods, mothers at home with their children were within shouting distance of each other over the backyard fence. Wherever children congregated, mothers would gather, too. There was ample opportunity for mothers to share the trials and tribulations of parenting. Mothers had each other for adult companionship and encouragement during the course of a long week with young children. Although our mothers may not have had the opportunity for a career outside the home — if they wanted one — they had each other. One important consequence of this social network was that when a mother gave birth to a new baby or was ill or needed any kind of assistance, other women would rally to help, bringing in meals, taking care of the older children, and helping out with the laundry or groceries.

Today, the woman who brings a new baby home from the hospital is in all likelihood someone with a career who is on a short maternity leave and doesn't even know her neighbors well. Few mothers will find their streets filled with other stay-at-home mothers who can drop by for coffee and some conversation. Her friends are mostly working women who will stop by with a baby gift but not have the time to bring home-cooked food or stay for the afternoon and help with the cleaning. Because our society is so transient, many women with new babies live far from their own mothers and can only enjoy perhaps a week-long visit from their mothers.

> *My mother is not a nurturing-type person. After I had my baby she gave me money to hire someone to help me. But I still didn't get the help I needed in picking up my older child, doing grocery shopping, that sort of thing . . . I was very ashamed to ask for help but I knew I was not going to get help from my mom. So I asked a ladies' group at my synagogue if they would help out. These people really fell through. I felt very betrayed, very hurt. One lady who did come over to help had so much resentment about it. I couldn't understand the purpose of this "sisterhood." I felt really crushed. I felt I had been dumped. My self-esteem just went down.*

The lack of female support and companionship is a serious handicap for today's new mothers. "In Western culture all too often there is a home, one woman, several small children and not enough female interdependence to share the heavy burden," says author Jane Price. "The concept of the nuclear family separates women, often leaving them alone with more child-care than one adult could reasonably be expected to cope."

MOTHERWORK

If you've been in this typical situation, you may have found the lack of support depressing or frightening. Your attempt to do everything without help or encouragement can be fulfilling in the short run (and is often applauded by society) but can lead to long-term fatigue and resentment. When you have a new baby, it's natural to want to do everything and prove your value as a mother. But why should you shoulder all of the responsibility?

> *As soon as I stepped foot in the house with the new baby, I felt totally overwhelmed. The logistics of getting two babies and two car seats into the car and getting out of the house overwhelmed me. I would sit there and think "In two more hours I have to do this." Seven weeks after my baby was born my older child had to have tubes in his ears. My husband also needed outpatient surgery. I felt completely unsupported and that no one was helping me.*

Postpartum depression, like burnout, may be a response to the organization of work — that is, having too much to do and not enough help. "Not all professionals have emotional problems; nor do all mothers. But there are times in any worker's life when job demands deplete, exhaust, and undermine. Motherwork, especially in relation to an infant, is a job of high demands," says Harriett Rosenberg, author of a chapter in the book *Feminism and Political Economy.*

> *My children were nineteen months apart. I felt from the moment I set foot in the house with the new baby that I was being buried under work. I was constantly picking things up, washing, holding a child, or preparing food or a bottle. Someone was always crying. By the end of the day, my back felt like it was going to break. I hated every moment of it. I didn't enjoy my youngest child as an infant. I didn't have the time.*

Motherwork generally involves a dependency on a husband (for income), on children (whose schedules set the day), and on experts for advice. You may feel you have very little control over your day. And at the end of the day, you may wonder what kind of contribution you've made to the world. Certainly few mothers ever hear anyone tell them, "Gee, you're a terrific mother. I can't believe how you play so cheerfully with your children, fix three meals a day, clean, and do the laundry — all so efficiently!"

> *I know exactly why I didn't get postpartum depression. I bought my way out. We hired a housekeeper to come in five days a week, make meals, clean, and babysit. I went out and just sat in the library. Eventually, I got a job and felt less guilty about the housekeeper.*

In past decades, there seemed to be more emotional support for new mothers. Society approved and applauded its new members. Assistance and advice to new mothers was always available. Children were highly valued.

Western cultures still contend that a new life is to be cherished and celebrated, but in reality, there are few support structures that take children into consideration. The lack of day-care alternatives for working mothers is one example. Moreover, new mothers may be penalized in the workplace. According to the Equal Employment Opportunity Commission, cases of pregnancy discrimination rose 7 percent from 1985 to 1990. Women taking maternity leave were more than 10 times more likely to lose their jobs than employees on other kinds of leaves.

With the signing of the 1992 Family and Medical Leave Act, women who work for employers with at least fifty employees are now entitled to take a twelve-week leave without fear of losing their jobs. However, this new legislation only specifies an unpaid leave. While some women are lucky enough to work for companies that offer a fully paid maternity leave, many others receive only partial pay, and many more receive no pay at all. In 1997, a study on the repercussions of the Family and Medical Leave Act found that most women were not taking full advantage of it because they could not afford to lose the income. In contrast, women in Scandinavian countries receive one or two *years* of parental leave at 90 percent of their salary.

"It is barbarous that a woman's right to as little as six weeks with her infant should even be open to argument. A truly civilized society would not use poverty or career penalties to blackmail women into leaving infants who are scarcely settled into life outside wombs that are still bleeding," says British psychologist Penelope Leach.

Even though most women will not lose their jobs for taking a modest maternity leave, employers still seem to feel that mothers are less committed employees. Many women returning to work find that they are no longer considered for special projects and promotions, and are encouraged to take a less responsible role than they had previously. On the flip side, some women complain that their employers have unrealistic expectations. More than one woman has returned to work on a part-time basis only to find that her employer expects her to accomplish as much as she used to when she was working full-time.

These circumstances pressure women to sometimes lie to others about parenting demands, hide their personal concerns from employers, and feel they have less right to flourish at work because they are mothers. Women tend to take the sole responsibility for the decision to become pregnant, and thus accept the "consequences." Given this lack of support, high demands, and high expectations, it's easy to see why many new mothers experience periods of frustration, exhaustion, and self-doubt.

Stress and the inability to admit that you are feeling stressed, angry, or unhappy are major factors in postpartum depression, according to Dr. Michael W. O'Hara, a University of Iowa researcher. O'Hara says women reporting more stressful life events and less support from spouses had higher rates of postpartum depression. Many depressed mothers reported difficulty in expressing their feelings to their spouses.

For two months I coped with it. My thoughts become darker. At times, I didn't want to go near my child. But I tried to act like everything was fine. Eventually, I broke down and told my husband how depressed I was. He didn't understand. He told me an idle mind is the devil's workshop.

You should recognize the difficult role society thrusts on you to combat depression and thrive. To offset these outside pressures, pay very close attention to your own needs. Here are some suggestions on how to do this:

- Be kind to yourself. Don't try to shoulder it all.
- Give yourself positive messages of praise and encouragement.
- Find a mothers group (it could be a postpartum illness support group, breastfeeding group, or play group) and encourage each other.
- Don't allow your employer to make you feel guilty about your parenting demands. Be assertive and press for changes in your workplace, such as parental leave and use of sick days to care for sick children or family emergencies.

If you're receiving therapy for postpartum depression or anxiety, you, your spouse, and your therapist should discuss motherwork and childrearing tasks. This aspect of postpartum depression is not an individual's problem but one in which society bears some responsibility. The problem is bigger than just you. Talking about it is the first step toward change.

MOTHERING IN OTHER CULTURES

We need only to look at societies that support and care lovingly for new mothers and their infants to see how postpartum psychiatric disorders might be alleviated or diminished for many women. In

Western cultures, the focus of childbirth is on the baby, the doctor, and the technology of the birth. However, in some tribal and agricultural societies, the focus is on the mother, and the extended family plays a central role. It is a custom that the new mother is surrounded by many helping hands. Let's look at a tribal society in Kenya that was studied by Sara Harkness of the Harvard School of Public Health.

In the Kipsigis community in Kenya, Harkness found no postpartum depression, which suggests that the culture is a powerful mediating factor between the physiological processes related to childbirth and their psychological outcomes. The Kipsigis are a traditional tribe with sex-segregated activities. Large families are desired. Pregnant women carry on with their tasks, and no public comment or preparation is made for the birth, which may be an attempt to protect the mother from too high expectations or some sad event such as the birth of a stillborn child.

Many women in the community attend the birth. The new mother receives special attention and has restrictions placed on her activities after the birth. The mother rests for at least seven days with restricted visitors. Other women cook, care for the other children, and clean, perhaps allowing the new mother to feel free to be emotionally dependent.

The father of the new baby is not allowed to see the child but provides goods for the baby and brings special food to help restore his wife's health. The mother usually returns to her tasks at about one month postpartum with her baby swaddled into a carrier on her back. The mother and the baby remain the center of attention. A party is held sometime after the baby is one month old to honor the family with gifts.[1]

This kind of society might help cushion a woman from postpartum depression. These women could not comprehend crying after birth. They saw birth as an entirely happy event.

In some cultures, childbirth as a physiological event is not as important as childbirth as a social event in that it confers a new role and status on a person or persons. Some researchers suggest that there are six elements in a society's structuring of the postpartum period that may help reduce the incidence of depression. These include:

1. A cultural recognition of the period, when the normal duties of the mother are interrupted
2. Protective measures designed to reflect the vulnerability of the new mother
3. Social seclusion
4. Mandated rest
5. Assistance with tasks
6. Social recognition of the new status for the mother through rituals, gifts, or other means

For example, in rural Guatemala, new mothers are considered very weak and delicate for eight days following childbirth, during which time they are kept resting and warm. And other cultures confer a period of a week or more of confinement and rest for a new mother, during which time she is explicitly cared for and is as much a center of concern and attention as is the new baby.[2]

Mothering Our Mothers

The birth of my daughter was normal, and I felt good during the thirty-six hours I spent in the hospital. But shortly after I took my baby home, she became jaundiced and had to be admitted to a children's hospital. At that hospital, parents are encouraged to stay with their children and help care for them, which I wanted to do. Yet I couldn't help but think how much easier it would have been for both my daughter and I if the jaundice had been detected and treated before we left the hospital where she was born. Instead, I spent twenty-four hours in the children's hospital with her, unable to eat or sleep because the hospital cafeteria was closed on Sundays and because there was no bed. My husband could not relieve me because he was at home with our three-year-old. When my daughter was discharged, I took her home and then went out to buy formula. As I stood in a checkout line to pay for the formula, I couldn't believe how much running around I had done despite having given birth only four days before. I was so tired I felt like collapsing.

The postpartum period is a time of particular vulnerability for a family. This vulnerability could manifest itself in postpartum depression, child abuse, or marital strife.

The solution to curbing the high incidence of postpartum depression might be as simple as learning to love and cherish parents, says Jane Honikman, president of Postpartum Support International (PSI) and a parent support volunteer with the Santa Barbara Birth Resource Center. "If only we would relearn the art of mothering our mothers. Other cultures do so with grace and dignity. They understand the fundamental necessity of having a well woman to nurture her family. At the same time, our fathers who have been thrust into the act of equal partner need to be supported, too."

MINORITY MOTHERS

The lack of social support for new mothers may be especially critical for minority women in the United States who come from different cultures and yet must adapt to a lifestyle of isolation and independence. If you are an immigrant and are coping with overwhelming problems, sadness, or anxiety, look for opportunities to be with other mothers in your community for companionship. Local community groups or centers may have free programs that will put you in touch with other mothers. One Los Angeles program for isolated, immigrant mothers was organized around a Head Start program. While the children met at Head Start, the mothers met in an adjacent classroom and discussed any topics they wanted. The sessions were free. Another place to look for some support is at local hospitals, where free programs are sometimes offered to parents who are adjusting to a new baby. If you're seeking a therapist, try to select one who is familiar with your ethnicity and culture.

LOW SUPPORT AND HIGH DEMANDS

As new mothers, we must resist society's unfair and uneducated expectations of us. Some observers would argue that as support for the mother role in our society has deteriorated, the workload mothers are expected to carry has soared.

In the last half of the twentieth century, it remains popular to believe that a child's well-being rests solely and squarely on the shoulders of his or her mother and on no one else — not society and not the father. The mother is expected to be completely in tune to the child's needs. With the development of this idea came a slew of books from experts focusing on the child and how the mother should best care for the child. The consequences are that:

- Mothers are blamed when thing go wrong.
- Mothers try to live up to the high standards asked of them.
- Mothers lose sight of their own feelings.

> *I would do it so differently now. I didn't have anyone I felt I could share my feelings of inadequacy with. I finally hired a nanny to help me with the baby. She was really a support person. She was attentive to me. I thought at the time I was hiring her for my daughter, but looking back, I know it was for me.*

With the responsibility for the child heaped on the mother, the pressure to be perfect is intense. If you feel — as many mothers do — that you are not living up to your image of a good mother, it may be because society has created unrealistic standards for mothers. The solution is to overhaul the standards, not yourself.

But too often mothers are blamed, and blame themselves, when things go wrong. The myth goes something like this: Mothers are responsible for every lazy, delinquent, underachieving, spoiled person on earth. The mother was selfish, overbearing, loveless, and demanding.

Although many of the popular parenting books are valuable, they too can lead us to believe that we have to do everything right — that there is no room for flexibility or mistakes. However, what we really need is to be instilled with self-confidence, not more instructions on how to diaper, feed, and take the baby's temperature.

Setting too-high goals can leave you feeling as if you are always falling short. Try to shed this self-consciousness over what kind of mother you are. Take what good you can from parenting books and others' advice and don't worry about the rest. You know your child better than anyone else. Your confidence and love will go a long, long way.

THE DESTRUCTIVE SUPERWOMAN

In past decades, the all-sacrificing mother was often called a martyr. Today, society has replaced that outdated title with one that is more glamorous and positive but equally destructive: the superwoman.

Whether we call ourselves martyrs or superwomen, some of us come to believe that we must give entirely of ourselves when we become mothers. We seem to feel that our families cannot survive unless we shoulder most of the burden. The superwoman myth is harmful because it thrusts the success of the family on you instead of defining motherhood as a role that should be imbedded within a network of social and public support.

But doing it all means being left without enough time or energy to tend to our own needs. Moreover, by trying to be superwoman, we are setting up conditions under which we are likely to fail. Further, the need to be totally in control and responsive to a child can lead to guilty feelings when things go wrong, as they invariably do.

Many mothers love and nurture children to the best of their abilities and still fear they are bad mothers. We want to be eternally loving, accessible, energetic, and patient mothers. But this is impossible. Further, it's not necessary. Our children need good-enough parents, not perfect parents. Superwomen, however, want things to be perfect and are least likely to admit when things aren't going well and to ask for help.

> *Every problem I've ever had in my life I could deal with. I don't know why I couldn't deal with this . . . It's not that I've gone now from depression to joy. It's from depression to normalcy.*

"The myth of the 'supermom' has a profound effect. It causes women to judge themselves, their mothers and their friends in its terms and makes it very difficult for women to talk to each other about the reality of their experience," say experts from the Pacific Post Partum Support Society in their handbook, *Post Partum Depression and Anxiety.*

> *The baby was premature and, for the first few weeks, she slept all the time. I was Miss Suzy Homemaker whizzing through the house. Then at one-and-a-half months old, the baby started screaming. I felt, all of a sudden, I'm doing things wrong. I felt like I was going backward.*

THE STATUS OF BEING A MOTHER

When you're working outside the home or are caring for children at home, you may find that your title as mother is one that will earn you the least amount of reverence. Sometimes it's easy to get down on yourself because society can make you feel as if you contribute little. Too little attention is given to postpartum depression caused by these cultural factors.

One research team studied a group of forty-nine first-time mothers from upper- and middle-class backgrounds, asking the women to complete questionnaires. All the women said they planned and wanted their pregnancies. But only 61 percent felt really positive about being pregnant. Overall, nearly 40 percent of women had loss of self-esteem. The authors said the change in self-esteem was due to the mothers' change in body image, public attitudes toward their pregnancies, and social life changes. Even the comments made to a pregnant woman can erode self-esteem.

"Today's attitude toward the role of motherhood may not have advanced much beyond that held in the early 1900s when pregnant women were basically sequestered at home during their term of pregnancy. This limited social life may be the most difficult aspect from which to recover," the authors of the study noted.[3]

A woman's eroding self-esteem as her pregnancy progresses can have an insidious effect on her attitude toward herself, her pregnancy, and her baby. But there is another reason for the lowered self-esteem of women who become mothers. Mothers today are revered less because children are revered less. Children today are viewed by society with perhaps the lowest regard ever seen in modern times. They are too often considered a drain on resources — a burden. Most mothers with young children will admit to an unease in taking a fussy child into a store to do a quick errand, for fear of offending or bothering everyone, being told how to calm the child, and being subjected to stares and looks of disgust or even outright criticism: "Why would you bring an infant to the grocery store!"

Society downgrades motherhood with these kinds of messages: Mothers don't live in the real world. Mothering is something done in one's spare time. Women who are intelligent and educated also do something else. You can't be "only a mother."

A period for me of long days and short years, of dia-
pers, runny noses, earaches, more Little League
games than you could believe possible, tonsils and
those unscheduled races to the hospital emergency
room; Sunday school and church, hours of urging
homework, short chubby arms around your neck
and sticky kisses and experiencing bumpy
moments — not many, but a few — of feeling that I'd
never, ever be able to have fun again, and coping
with the feeling that [my husband], in his excite-
ment of starting a small company and traveling
around the world, was having a lot of fun.

You can see from this comment by former First Lady Barbara
Bush, from a 1985 speech reported in the *Los Angeles Times*, that
even women of social prestige and influence and wealth can feel
diminished by the way society views their contributions as mothers.
Even Britain's Princess Diana has revealed her struggles with postpartum depression.

Despite the choices it has created, some people feel the
women's movement has not done much to promote the self-esteem
of mothers. However, the women's movement has tried more in
recent years to present a more honest, realistic view of motherhood. The movement that has propelled more women than ever
before into political office can now demand that government promote family causes.

WORKING OUTSIDE THE HOME

For women who work outside the home, society's low regard for
the role of mother and the welfare of children is especially problematic. About 65 percent of women with children under eighteen
are in the work force, according to 9 to 5, the National Association
of Working Women. Women who work outside the home may be
at higher risk of depression than their stay-at-home counterparts,

according to some studies.[4] It seems having a paycheck and a career don't buffer you from the pressures of hard work.

You may have viewed your own mother as being "trapped" at home and thwarted from self-expression and freedom. Perhaps you vowed to have a different kind of life, one with more choices. Indeed, women growing up in the 1960s and 1970s had more opportunities to break from the mold: to opt for work and opt out of motherhood. But our rejection of our mothers' lives has led to guilt. Women tend to feel guilty about working when their own mothers devoted themselves to the children. The guilt is that "I'm not fulfilling what I should be doing as a mother," says Barbara J. Berg, author of the book *The Crisis of the Working Mother.*

"It is important to be absolutely clear about this — the guilt does not originate in the dual pursuit of career and motherhood. The specific tasks of coordinating both roles — the logistics of it — provide our unconscious guilt with a perfect opportunity to attach itself. With magnetic tenacity, guilt adheres to the issues surrounding the combination of work and mothering. But it arises from the decision to be different from our mother, to choose a different lifestyle, to challenge her values, attitudes, child-rearing practices — this appears to conflict with what we have learned from our mother, with her standards of mothering, which are also our own." To resolve this conflict and soothe guilt, many women absorb this societal message: It's okay if you want to work as long as you don't ignore your family and home.

I used to work as a professional in the school system. But I don't feel I have a lot to offer right now.

Few mothers find the choice of whether or not to work outside the home easy. Society hands out conflicting messages to the new mother about both. If you work outside the home, you are neglecting your family. If you work raising children at home, you are of little interest to society. Given this double-edged sword, plus the pressure from husbands and parents and financial considerations, how many women are really free to do what they want to do? How many feel ambivalent about their choice?

Women who work outside the home face the complications of carrying out multiple roles. Studies show that many couples feel the dual roles create more stress than they would prefer. If the male partner approves of the woman's choices with regard to working outside or inside the home, he is more likely to help out and be supportive and the stress on her is eased somewhat. Also, women with child care problems or who are dissatisfied with child care are more stressed out.

It's not always possible to choose the way we would most like to spend our time. In fact, it's rare that anyone has that choice! The trick, in terms of your mental well-being, is to come to terms with what you want, how you feel, and what you're doing. Ask yourself these questions in order to clarify how your work status or role may affect your emotions:

- Are you doing what you always envisioned or dreamed you would do after becoming a mother? (In other words, did you think you would stay at home full-time and instead find you must work outside the home?)
- Do you gain satisfaction from what you do?
- Is your spouse supportive of what you are doing?
- Does your child (or children) seem happy and well cared for?
- Do you feel good about your child care?
- Do you feel you are rewarded and appreciated for what you do?

If your answer to most of these questions is "yes," chances are your depression has little to do with role strain. But if your answer to most of these questions is "no," you need to consider whether these areas are the primary source of your unhappiness and anxiety. These are most definitely topics to discuss in therapy. Although you may not be able to change the "big picture," like your employment status, you can usually influence the circumstances around you to alleviate some of the stress.

OUTSIDE WORK AND CHILDREN

The good news is that recent research shows it is not harmful to children when both parents work outside the home. Good child care — a clean, safe place with consistency in the staff and a proper teacher-to-child ratio — has not been linked to any developmental problems in children. Moreover, studies find children flourish when they receive love and attention from several adults. Quality day care often enhances a child's social and cognitive development. And working mothers set good role models for their children while breaking down sex stereotypes that have held women back. Mothers shouldn't think they are the only ones who can care adequately for children. Children need love, support, acceptance, and affirmation from fathers, relatives, friends, and society.

Indeed, the real problem may lie with how both parents feel and respond to the day care arrangement. If the mother is sad and guilty and the father is unhappy, a child may pick up on that. Guilt changes the way we react to our children. We might be more likely to overcompensate for absences, insist on quality time, change the way we discipline, and expect less of our children.

Women who work outside the home might be better prepared to handle the complexities of their roles if they earned good wages and could thus afford to hire the help they need to care for their homes and families. But 80 percent of all working women are still in traditional women's jobs with low wages and low status: for example, waitresses, file clerks, and hospital aides. The average weekly salary for these types of jobs is $328, while men in similar jobs earn $468, according to one study.[5]

Moreover, the business world, for the most part, has shown little interest in helping working mothers meet both home and job obligations. Few employers have felt it necessary to supply adequate child care programs; explore part-time, flexible-time, and job-sharing programs; or offer extended maternity leave or time off to care for a sick child. In fact, 50 percent of all working mothers in the United States have no maternity leave benefit.[6]

The burden of the working mother cannot be underestimated as a factor in depression. In many cases, a mother returns to work only six weeks after having her child.

> *I knew my maternity leave would be the only long period that I would have to devote entirely to my baby. My boss told me I had to return at the end of my six-week leave or he could not hold my job open. The Sunday before I returned, I cried off and on all day. I looked at that tiny baby and wondered what would happen. Would he think I had abandoned him? Would the sitter take good care of him? I was leaving him with a virtual stranger. I felt torn, and I still do.*

Well, that's a heavy dose of reality to swallow, and it's more than anyone can tackle alone. The point is to remember that postpartum illness can be a response to the world we live in — one that asks much of mothers. A new philosophy in treating this kind of depression centers on exploring these social factors and finding ways to overcome them. In other words, this kind of depression can be "good," or even healthy, if it helps you to identify areas of strain in your life and make positive changes. The process starts by looking at what is causing your unhappiness, what you can change, and what you can learn to live with. Does your workplace offer flexible working arrangements, such as part-time work? Could you transfer to a department where there is a supervisor who is more understanding of the pressures on working parents? If you work at home, could you join a mother's group or take classes to provide sources of companionship, support, and fun? Are there better day-care arrangements that would make you feel more confident? Can you and your spouse better divide the child care and household tasks?

It takes some time and courage to make changes like these. However, they can make a big difference in your emotional health.

CHAPTER FIVE

Other Risk Factors

On December 25, 1993, my husband and I were blessed with a special gift, a perfect baby girl on Christmas Day. I had no prior history of psychiatric illness and had an uneventful and easy pregnancy. I guess I have always had difficulty understanding why this happened to me. What put me at such greater risk?

Women who suffer from a postpartum mood disorder will invariably ask "Why me? Why did this happen to me?" Usually, this is not a question with a clearcut answer. Certainly some women seem to be affected more by hormonal changes after childbirth. Others have clear stresses in their lives that can trigger depression — such as the case of a woman whose mother died just weeks before she gave birth to her first child. But quite often, postpartum illness is the result of a collision of many factors that can include hormonal changes, the negative societal conditions affecting new mothers, and individual stressors. That is why the illness is sometimes called a multifactorial disorder.

In addition to the sweeping explanations of hormones and societal conditions, experts have singled out several risk factors that are frequently associated with postpartum illness. These factors are discussed in the following sections.

PERSONAL OR FAMILY HISTORY OF MENTAL ILLNESS

Joan is a tiny, fair woman with two daughters. Recently, she began to recover from years of psychiatric illness — both depression and psychosis. While her illness became apparent shortly after the birth of her first child, Joan feels she has battled depression most of her life and that the births of her two children sent her over the edge . . . "I feel I have been suffering from depression since I was a child. I had learning disabilities and had to stay back and repeat the second grade. I always had such low self-esteem. I wasn't able to get into college because of my grades. So, when I was nineteen, I took up dance. That was something I clung to because I liked it so much. But the competition was so strong I gave up trying to make it as a dancer. It was like a shattered dream. I seemed to get more depressed after that. I also had premenstrual tension syndrome. I always had trouble with my periods and became so depressed with the PMS." Joan married her teen-age sweetheart and they had a baby shortly after their marriage. The child was good-natured and Joan and her husband were thrilled. But, two weeks after the child's birth, Joan experienced the first of many black depressions.

A personal history of psychiatric illness is a red flag for postpartum psychiatric illness. In a 1985 study in Great Britain of mothers admitted to psychiatric units within twelve months of childbirth, 34 out of 142 mothers had a past history of psychosis, and an additional 23 had experienced a nonpsychotic mental illness in the past.[1] Another study found that women previously diagnosed with a bipolar depressive illness have a 30 to 40 percent chance of having a depression in the postpartum period.[2]

What is it about childbirth that triggers another bout of a psychiatric illness? Hormones may be the cause. The stress of having a new baby could play a role. Any medical disorder, such as anemia, hyperthyroidism, or diabetes can be exacerbated when an individual is under extreme stress. "Depression, panic disorder, obsessive-compulsive disorder — all these are illnesses we believe to be caused by abnormalities of chemicals in the brain, probably hereditary, but also made worse by stress and psychosocial factors," says Dr. Deborah Hines, a physician and postpartum expert in St. Louis, Missouri.

Women who have suffered from a mental health problem in the past often look to pregnancy and childbirth as joyous events that might help them feel normal and happy. Unfortunately, they remain at high risk for a relapse after childbirth.

Because depression is a disease with genetic, or hereditary, underpinnings, a family history of psychiatric illness can increase a woman's risk of suffering a postpartum disorder.

Finally, depression during the pregnancy, which is relatively uncommon, increases the risk of postpartum depression. Two things are important here: (1) Prevention efforts must include a review of a woman's psychiatric past. Every woman in prenatal care should be asked about her mental health history. (2) If you are in therapy for postpartum depression and have also had past mental health problems, your therapy should have a broader focus than just issues surrounding childbirth. Your therapy should include a plan to prevent relapse of the disorder.

REPRODUCTIVE HISTORY

Will having a healthy, full-term infant stir up negative feelings if you've had an abortion, miscarriage, or stillbirth, perhaps contributing or causing postpartum depression? That question is debated, especially where abortion is concerned. One out of every three pregnancies ends in abortion. That leaves a large population of women with some history of abortion who may later carry a full-term pregnancy.

One British study found that depression was highly correlated with a history of abortion but not with miscarriage. The authors of the study suggested that the depression was a manifestation of dormant grief. The women in the study frequently expressed worries that the baby might be born damaged. Many mothers also felt that if the baby was born with some health problem, it would signal that the mother was being punished for the abortion.[3]

But even though a strong myth prevails that women who have abortions harbor long-term guilt and anxiety, that finding has not been borne out scientifically. Most studies, including more recent studies, fail to show a long-term psychological response to abortion. According to a 1990 study by a University of New York at Buffalo psychologist, few women undergoing first-trimester abortions in the United States suffer severe negative psychological reactions. "The predominant response to such an abortion experience is relief. Feelings of depression, regret, and guilt may also be experienced after the procedure, but they are typically mild and transitory and do not affect general functioning," the study reported.[4]

Psychological response to abortion, however, varies among women. It can relate to age, reason for the abortion, past mental health history, the actual abortion procedure, and expressions of social support or disapproval.

Past miscarriages and stillbirths are also events that might become important in the postpartum period, even if you've just borne a healthy child. It's normal that the birth of a child would revive some unresolved grief over lost pregnancies. Sometimes it is not until a woman bears a healthy child that the loss of another infant is fully realized.

If you have not discussed the loss of a previous pregnancy, the best thing you can do is to talk it out. A recent Columbia University study found that women who miscarried and spoke for ninety minutes to three hours on the phone with a nonmedical hospital worker two weeks after their loss were substantially less depressed when they were interviewed again four weeks later. But women who did not speak with a hospital worker after miscarriage were found to be more depressed six weeks later. Four months later, neither group was more depressed than other women. The authors of the study urge women to meet with their obstetricians (and the obstetrician should encourage the patient to come in) to discuss the miscarriage.[5] But it may not matter too much who you talk to about this as long as that person listens carefully and provides support.

Abortions, miscarriages, and stillbirths are not the only events in a woman's reproductive history that can become important in the postpartum period. Infertility also is a major cause of depression among young women. And although infertility is frequently overcome to produce a full-term pregnancy, some women (and men) are surprised to find they still face lingering feelings of depression that stem from the infertile phase of their lives.

> I think, after infertility, you expect every moment is going to be perfect. You've waited for this baby for so long. After five years of infertility, I wanted to be the most perfect mother. Not too long ago we wouldn't even have been able to have a child.

Infertility can become identified as the cause of a woman's unhappiness and prevent her from facing and dealing with other problems in her life, says Dr. Elizabeth Herz in *Postpartum Psychiatric Illness*. To expect all her unhappiness or problems would disappear with the arrival of a baby (through birth or adoption) is unrealistic and sets the mother up for serious disappointment. "The realization of previously unacknowledged problems together with the disappointment of her unrealistic expectations can put a woman into a tailspin of depression," she says.

The recovery process here also begins with acknowledging unresolved feelings and discussing them. A good place to start may be the infertility support group Resolve. This national group has hundreds of local chapters (see the Resources section), where you can meet other couples who may share your experiences. Don't be afraid to attend the meetings even if you've already had or adopted a baby. The group helps couples in all phases of infertility (even post-infertility) work through issues aggravated by years of infertility.

Pregnancy and the Birth Experience

Pregnancy and childbirth are events that create such high expectations, you may wonder if problems or disappointments associated with these events can cause postpartum depression. Studies are mixed on this point. In some studies, a difficult pregnancy or birth experience was not found to be linked to postpartum depression, probably because a woman receives extra support when she is ill compared with a woman who breezes through her pregnancy and childbirth.[6]

But other studies have shown instances where the birth experience does appear to contribute to postpartum depression. According to experts from the Pacific Post Partum Support Society, the birth experience may be a factor, but is highly unlikely, by itself, to be the cause of postpartum depression.

Although rare, pregnancy can be a time of increased vulnerability to depression for some women. Little attention is usually paid to a woman's feelings, moods, and thoughts at this time. During pregnancy you probably experienced heightened emotions: tearfulness, irritability, anxiety, for example. Excitement and happiness are sometimes sabotaged by fear and worry — about the health of the baby, about labor and delivery, about how you will hold up as a mother, or about how your life will change after the baby. Even the physical aspects of pregnancy — fatigue, nausea, weight gain, and loss of sexual attractiveness — can take their toll.

But although pregnancy is always emotional, what is psychologically normal or abnormal about it has not been well defined.

Depression might be a factor during the pregnancy and postpartum if you had doubts or were ambivalent about having a baby. Likewise, the father's negative reaction to the pregnancy can cause depression in the mother-to-be. "Reactions of both parents to the pregnancy is very important," says Tamara Ostapowicz, a St. Louis, Missouri obstetrician. "We've had a number of couples where . . . the father is not as involved and not as supportive of the pregnancy." For example, in one case a woman underwent a prenatal blood test for a common birth defect. The test showed ambiguous results, and physicians recommended the woman undergo amniocentesis, a more reliable prenatal test. But the woman did not undergo the amniocentesis because of her husband's ambivalence about the test. She then endured six months of anxiety wondering if the baby had a birth defect.

Sometimes, it can seem as if the depression or psychosis arises out of the very birth experience. Experiences that have been considered as factors in depression include having a cesarean section, the unanticipated use of anesthesia, stillbirth, and multiple birth.

Some studies indicate that having a cesarean section is a factor in postpartum illness, but other studies do not support this. One found that a stressful delivery is associated with a lower frequency of postpartum depression. This, again, may be because the new mother is afforded additional support, attention, and reassurance.[7]

The anxiety and pain of labor is seldom mentioned as a contributing factor in postpartum illness. But having support and preparation for childbirth might play a preventive role. According to an interesting article in the 1980 edition of the *New England Journal of Medicine,* the effects of a supportive person (called a *doula*) on the length of labor and on mother-infant interaction after delivery were significant. The authors found that in all but 1 of 150 cultures studied by anthropologists, a family member or friend, usually a woman, remained with the mother during labor and delivery.[8] The message from this study seems to be that support and companionship during birth is important and that these effects may endure well beyond labor and delivery. This may be particularly important to the single woman bearing a child, especially teen-age mothers.

Preconceived notions of what the birth will (or should) be like often set women up for disappointments that can become a contributing factor to the emergence of postpartum illness. Although well-prepared childbirth classes and books have been instrumental in encouraging couples to expand their options, take control, and seek what they want in childbirth, the philosophy is all too often rigid and implies that if there are surprises at birth, then the couple has done something wrong. Mothers are often especially disheartened and guilt-ridden when they end up with a cesarean section.

For some women, the abrupt shift from being the center of attention during the pregnancy to the baby's becoming the focus of attention is depressing. "Another person — the baby — comes on the scene to garner attention just when the mother herself is most at need both physically and emotionally," says K. C. Cole, the author of the book *What Only a Mother Can Tell You About Having a Baby.* "Birth makes you irrelevant. Now the subject of everyone's affections and attentions is the new baby. Not that nobody cares about you. Of course they do. But you're no longer the main attraction. The trouble is that the body and mind you've been nursing so carefully for so many months hasn't gone away. And it still has a lot of recovering to do."

"The way we catapult mothers now out of the hospital after giving birth, we're not even able to pick up the onset of blues," says Dr. Deborah Sichel, clinical instructor in psychiatry at Harvard Medical School. "So we send a mother out, back into her home, with no support. She hasn't even established a breast milk supply. She hasn't even learned how to start being the care giver and we've catapulted her out of the hospital."

Much can be done to address these kinds of risk factors. If you've had a disappointing birth experience, talk it out as soon as possible with your spouse, mother, friend, or doctor. Work through it right away so that you can focus on what's ahead of you — not what's behind you. In addition, arriving home from the hospital much more sore, tired, anxious, and frazzled than you expected is a surefire signal that you may need more help for the next few weeks. Not feeling well is always worse when you expected to feel fine!

STRESSFUL LIFE EVENTS

> *This baby was with my second husband, and we hadn't been married that long. My first child was born eleven years ago. So there was this big age gap. I kept thinking, "Here I am, starting all over again." I had also had a miscarriage six months before.*

Studies have repeatedly shown that stressful life events often contribute to postpartum disorders. The major predictors of postpartum blues are family and personal history of depression, stressful life events, and social adjustment, according to one study.[9]

"Despite the fact that pregnancy is clearly a huge stressor, the onset of other kinds of things in terms of a woman's life [can be a factor], such as perhaps moving, losing a job, starting a new job, starting a new course at school, taking exams," Sichel says. "It's really surprising to me today how much women actually take on at the time of pregnancy. I see people doing the bar exam. And very often women will move during a pregnancy and then will be in a new neighborhood not knowing anybody and not having any kind of social support . . . It's very important for women to be counseled not to make major decisions and major moves . . . during that period."

Other stressors can include the loss of a parent, a poor relationship with a parent, financial problems, concern for other children, inadequate household help, and inadequate housing. Some women do not feel comfortable bringing a new baby into their current living environment. They may feel unsafe in their house, apartment, or neighborhood.

If you've had outside stresses around the time of childbirth, recognize that these may have contributed to your negative feelings. Try not to take on anything extra. Call a halt to the party you've planned in four weeks (and thought you'd feel good enough to host). Try to put ongoing problems, such as financial strains, on the back burner for at least a portion of every day to focus solely on yourself and your baby. Obviously, dealing with the source of your stress is imperative. If you can't deal with the circumstances at the moment, escape for awhile. Move in with a friend or relative or try to find a temporary solution to your problems. Ask for help and advice from others. You deserve and need extra support right now. Seek counseling on how to take concrete steps toward a solution.

BREASTFEEDING

Breastfeeding can also become a very stressful situation in the life of a new mother. Again, breastfeeding can be a factor in postpartum depression but probably is not the only cause, experts say. Breastfeeding, while very rewarding and satisfying to most women (and easy for many), can also be fatiguing, stressful, and frustrating. It can also prevent the father from taking a more active, helpful role during the postpartum period.

> *By the time my daughter was two-and-a-half weeks old, I was put in therapy and on medication for depression and abruptly stopped breastfeeding. This was a huge relief to me because it calmed me down. Plus, I hadn't enjoyed breastfeeding at all since I felt such a lack of attachment. I felt very guilty about this since I had always planned to*

breastfeed. I do hope I will be able to when I have a second child.

Breastfeeding is yet another experience that can produce guilt and anxiety in a new mother when things don't go well. You may feel you should breastfeed because it's often recommended, but you may feel anxious or uncomfortable about it.

You call breastfeeding experts for help and they say, "Whatever you do, don't stop breastfeeding." They totally neglect the mother. They forget that the healthy mother means a healthy child.

Breastfeeding can be an additional, unnecessary burden if you have other risk factors for postpartum illness. "Mothers are often made to feel that they are responsible for the success of breastfeeding as if it is something that good mothers know how to do and then enforce on the baby," says Jane Price, the author of *Motherhood: What It Does to Your Mind.* "Like so much of motherhood there is a suggestion that if the mother gets it right the baby will go along unquestioningly with her."

The lack of preparation, poor teaching methods, and high expectations are to blame when breastfeeding fails. A government study found that a majority of physicians in obstetrics, gynecology, pediatrics, and general practice are not prepared to offer women effective counseling and support on breastfeeding.[10] But women blame themselves for failure. Again, the ideal and reality conflict, and the hapless new mother is the victim.

This can lead to resentment and anger and a pattern of self-sacrifice and self-denial. Physically and psychologically, breastfeeding is best for the baby. But remember that your own preferences and limitations, as well as your environment, should be taken into account. If you do encounter problems but want to continue breastfeeding, the key is to act fast. Call your pediatrician and ask for a referral to a lactation consultant. These consultations can usually be arranged at your home within four to twenty-four hours, and your health insurance may cover part of the $30 to $70 per hour cost of the consultation. (See the Resources section for lactation organizations.) One lactation organization, the La Leche League, is a wonderful free service for new mothers. Members can give you immediate help — or a referral to a professional — and can provide ongoing, long-term support. (Consult your phone book for a chapter near you.)

Finally, remember to ask your "buffers" — your spouse or a relative — to honor and protect your need for peace and quiet as you learn to breastfeed your baby. And if it's too much, give it up. Only you can decide when the benefits of breastfeeding are no longer worth what it is costing you. Your baby will thrive on formula, and you can rest assured that you've made the right decision because it's your decision.

THE SICK OR DIFFICULT CHILD

Having an infant who is premature, sick, colicky, a poor sleeper, or frequently fussy constitutes an important risk factor for depression. It is little wonder new mothers often discuss among themselves whether the newborn is a "good baby"; they are acknowledging how important the baby's temperament is to their own well-being. According to experts, difficult or sick babies are factors in postpartum illness but are unlikely to be the sole cause.

> *The health problem has been an added stress . . . seeing doctors all the time and planning her surgery. But I don't know if I would have had this [depression] anyway, without this added stress.*

One issue new parents with a sick or difficult infant face is that they question whether their parenting skills are at fault. Nothing can bring a new mother to tears faster than hearing how "easy" a friend's baby is while her own cries or fusses most of the day. Likewise, it is a stab of sorrow for the parent of a baby with a physical or mental handicap or illness to hear of all the "perfect" babies being born to those around them.

> *I was convinced that her small size was due to a medical problem or somehow my fault. I'm prone to worrying, and I grew up in a troubled family. And I'm sure those things played a part in the particular manifestation of my depression. At any rate, the notion that I may have caused some problem that my daughter might possibly have was almost more than I could bear, yet was something that I couldn't shake from my mind.*

Mothers might also become depressed about an ill child simply because they are unable to care for and nurture the infant the way they had anticipated during pregnancy. Premature or very ill newborns are whisked off to intensive care units and parents might have to wait weeks before they can even hold their babies.

Even mothers with healthy but temperamentally difficult infants find themselves comparing their lives with those of other mothers. Studies have found infant temperament was a significant risk factor for stress in depressed women. "Babies vary a great deal. Some are more demanding and difficult to care for than others. Whether your infant is difficult or easy makes a great difference if you are depressed," says Donna Gelfant, a University of Utah expert on postpartum illness.

One way to reduce postpartum depression may be to arm yourself with more parenting skills — such as those acquired by a mother who has already had a baby or two. You've probably heard parents talk about how much easier their second child is. That may be because they've learned many good parenting skills that make things easier.

> *When she screams and cries I feel so bad because I can't do anything to help her. I took her to the store the other day and she was screaming and everyone was*

*looking at me like "What are you doing to her?" . . .
Every time I went to the doctor I'd feel like an idiot
because I was complaining about her crying and she
was so sweet and good in the office.*

Nothing can rattle a parent more than the incessant crying of a newborn. For mothers who are already blue or depressed, excessive crying can send them over the edge. Moreover, studies of child battering show that sick or handicapped children are more likely to be spanked or abused — most likely because they are difficult to care for and lead parents who are already coping poorly to snap.

Many babies go through a colicky period for weeks or months. Colic attacks usually occur in the late afternoon and evening when parents are most tired. Colic is poorly understood by medical professionals, which is a shame because it causes more misery to the parents of infants than practically any other medical condition. A long-held explanation is that colic is caused by excessive gas or disturbances in the infant's intestines. Sometimes, changing an infant's formula and the use of prescription or over-the-counter medications for gas can help. Other doctors suggest that colic is simply a response to the infant's immature central nervous system and inability to adapt and become comfortable in his or her environment.

Another recent theory, suggested by Dr. Bruce Taubman, the author of studies on colic at Children's Hospital of Philadelphia's Division of Gastroenterology and Nutrition, is that colic is caused by the parents' well-intentioned mishandling of their baby's needs. For example, parents may assume that the baby is crying due to hunger or a wet diaper when the baby just wants to be held.

Whatever the cause, most parents find that colic can rock their family life.

"As with most situations affecting infants, infant colic syndrome is a family condition, involving everyone who lives in the household," says Taubman, author of the book *Curing Infant Colic: The 7-Minute Program for Soothing the Fussy Baby.* "Because it affects the family's sleep and because if unattended it can go on for months, infant colic syndrome can turn a family upside down and disrupt those first weeks in which parents and child get to know each other and establish their patterns of interaction."

Disappointment is a common reaction among parents with colicky infants, Taubman says. Excessive crying in infants elicits anxiety in parents. Physiologically, a crying child can cause its mother's heartbeat to speed up. She may also experience sweating, increased alertness, and even fear. When a mother's actions to deal with the crying fail, anxiety results. Parents can also experience sleep deprivation as a result of an infant's excessive crying, as well as guilt and disappointment in their relationship with the infant.

"Understand that you would not be human if you did not feel disappointed at your frustrated expectations," Taubman says. "Disappointment and dismay are universal reactions among parents of inconsolable babies. You may not be able to eliminate the sting of these emotions, but knowing their pervasiveness may keep you from experiencing guilt at having them."

Parents also tend to have these reactions to crying infants:

- I'm doing something wrong.
- I should never have had a baby. I'm not cut out for this.
- I want to run away.
- I'm making this baby cry for some reason.
- My baby senses I want to return to work.
- I'm the only mother who can't comfort her baby. My baby must not like me.
- I don't love the baby enough and he can tell.

If you have a colicky infant, you must take care of your own needs in order to respond appropriately to the baby. This might require the services of a babysitter for a period each day so that you or your husband can get a break from the child and catch up on sleep.

Seek help from your pediatrician to explore the reasons for the baby's crying. Prescription medication for colic is available. This mild sedative and gastrointestinal medication can help alleviate some crying. If your pediatrician refuses to prescribe it or tells you that nothing can be done to help your child, find a new pediatrician. Keep in close touch with your pediatrician for support and encouragement. If your doctor cannot provide this support, find another pediatrician.

If you're experiencing symptoms of blues or depression, consider hiring or enlisting full-time help while your spouse is working during the day. Some cities are opening special day care centers for children who are chronically ill or disabled, and these centers often take infants with colic. Inquire into day care for your infant to save yourself from the strain of the infant's excessive crying for at least part of each day. There will be plenty of time for you and your infant to re-establish a relationship when the your health has improved and when your baby's colic has abated.

POSTPARTUM FATIGUE

Postpartum fatigue has emerged in recent years as a significant problem for a segment of new mothers. According to one study, the two weeks following childbirth are the most critical for a new mom.[11] Fatigue and depressive thoughts are greatest during this time. The study found that the loss of sleep and infant care demands seem to peak at the two-week point. It is not clear whether the fatigue is caused by depression or whether depression causes fatigue. But there is no doubt that feeling or being tired can exacerbate depression.

Fatigue is an important risk factor in postpartum illness. According to Katharina Dalton, the British physician who has studied reproductive mood disorders extensively, postpartum fatigue can be a separate postpartum psychiatric disorder in addition to the others (such as blues, depression, and psychosis) commonly mentioned. Fatigue after childbirth can be a symptom of thyroid disorders, anemia, infections, cardiomyopathy, or mood disorders. If you are fatigued and not functioning on what should be enough sleep, ask your physician about having a thyroid test. Low thyroid hormone output can cause sluggishness and fatigue. Anemia, a common complication after childbirth, can also cause fatigue. Many obstetricians recommend new mothers continue taking prenatal vitamin supplements and iron tablets for a couple months after childbirth to counteract anemia.

Women often complain of sadness and irritability stemming from a birth that "took a lot out of me." This fatigue might actually be a mild form of depression. The fatigue can be physical or mental, healthy or unhealthy. Healthy fatigue comes from a day of rewarding output in which a woman feels satisfied with her day and sleeps soundly, waking rested. Or it can be an unhealthy tiredness that appears as mental dullness and the lack of energy. Lethargy is the dominant feature of this type of fatigue. The symptoms include wanting to sleep all the time and never getting enough sleep. Often, experts note, fatigue is insidious. Women may not recognize how exhausted they've become. Postpartum fatigue should be of concern when it becomes disabling, lasts more than six weeks past delivery, delays the resumption of normal activities, and impairs a patient's recovery, according to researchers.

STRENGTH OF THE MARRIAGE

The strength of the marriage is another important factor in whether a woman at risk for postpartum depression becomes ill and/or how easily she recovers. In general, studies show that marriage confers a greater protection against depression on men than women. In unhappy marriages, women are three times as likely as men to be depressed. In general, young married women are more likely to report sadness than married men or their single female peers.

A poor marital relationship is the most significant risk factor for postpartum depression, says Dr. Ricardo Fernandez, an assistant professor of clinical psychiatry at the Robert Woods Johnson/Rutgers Medical School. Problems in the marriage can be characterized by disappointment about the father's participation in child care, an inequitable breakdown of responsibilities and tasks in the home, and the husband being emotionally unavailable.

Maybe you're supposed to discuss all of this before the baby is born. But how do you know it's going to be like this?

Marriage problems can include poor communication, a conflictual relationship, being nonsupportive of each other, and a poor sexual relationship. Further, studies have found that women feel isolated and lonely when their marriages are based on relationships of inequality and emotional distance, report the authors of "Women and Depression," published by the American Psychological Association. This is especially common when the woman works outside the home and when there are children at home.

I think there is that kind of unspoken comment that "you're not the wife you were before."

Studies of working women have shown that when husbands helped with child and household care (and if the woman's employment was important to both partners' values and preferences), employment of the woman was associated with improved mental health. "But employment did not affect the mental health of women whose husbands did not help them with child care."[12]

If you believe the roots of your depression stem from marriage problems, seek help from a marriage and family therapist (along with your spouse, if possible). Having a child can sometimes exacerbate marital conflicts. But a baby can provide a good reason to clear the air and address your problems. Remember, too, that postpartum disorders often cause stress and strain on even the healthiest marriages. The marital conflicts may be a side effect from the illness. Sometimes it's hard to identify the real source of the trouble. But the roots of the problem will become more clear if you and your spouse seek and persist in getting professional counseling.

POVERTY AND SINGLE MOTHERS

I have no one to help me when she gets on my nerves. She was crying and fussing the whole day yesterday. I was totally tired and exhausted. I was trying to make dinner and it was totally impossible. She was so fussy. I thought I was going to go out of my mind.

The risk for postpartum illness is increased when a woman is a single parent, according to a British study.[13] Although not all single mothers have financial problems, a great many struggle to provide for a child on one income — especially those women with few job skills or little job experience whose partner or spouse leaves them unexpectedly. Thus, another risk factor for depression — poverty — might come into play.

Poverty is called "a pathway to depression" by experts at the American Psychological Association. According to these experts, studies show that inadequate income over a long period of time can lead to personal uncertainty, social isolation, and a high frequency of negative events. These things, in turn, lead to depression.

If you're raising a child alone, it's very important to surround yourself with supportive people. There are several good resources for single parents, including groups like Single Mothers by Choice, Parents Without Partners, and the Single Parents Resource Center. (See the Resources section in the back of this book for more information.) Many support groups for single parents are free, and you can bring your children.

PERSONALITY AND COPING STYLES

Your personality type — how you handle things — can contribute to the emergence of a postpartum illness. Women with depression were commonly found to have personality types of avoidant, passive, or dependent behavior, as well as exhibiting pessimistic and negative thinking styles. Research suggests women, especially women of this personality type, often focus too much on discussing depressed feelings instead of taking action to deal with them.

A need to be organized, always in control, and perfectionistic is another personality type that increases a woman's risk. "Some issues, such as inflexibility and control, may not have been a problem to the patient before her illness," says Fernandez in his textbook *Postpartum Psychiatric Illness*. "In fact, these highly organized women do quite well in the working world. However, the demands of raising a child require patience and acceptance of many things that cannot be rigidly controlled."

If this is your situation, you need not clobber yourself with blame for the way you are. Your strong personality traits no doubt serve you well in many ways. As for being a mother, classes that teach parenting skills may do you much good. You can learn to develop methods that expand your patience and tolerance. Check local schools, hospitals, churches, the YMCA, and community colleges for parenting classes. Information on parenting also is available through resource centers such as Mothers Matter and the National Association of Mothers' Centers. (See the Resources section in the back of this book for more information on these centers and for a list of some good parenting books.)

PAST VICTIMIZATION

If you have been a victim of emotional, physical, or sexual abuse, chances are high that this experience is playing some part in your illness. High rates of depression are common in women who have been victimized. Beware that medical professionals caring for women with postpartum depression sometimes overlook this as a risk factor. Your past victimization is something that needs to be addressed during your recovery.

Rose and Donald were married in 1986 after dating for several years. They were a happy, close couple. Rose was a company vice president of a family-owned business and Donald had a paint distributorship. The couple discussed having a baby for a few years after their marriage and, after a vacation in Canada, Rose became pregnant.

"To hear the words that I was pregnant was a shock. But as soon as I passed the nausea period, everything came together. We just had a blast decorating the nursery and having parties. Everyone treated me really special. I was one of those glowing people, and I was really happy. I couldn't wait for the baby," says Rose, a vivacious woman.

A baby boy was born to Rose and Donald in September, 1989. But from the moment of childbirth on, Rose began experiencing difficulties. Rose's contractions had come on quickly and strongly. Enduring intense labor pain, she wanted to begin pushing the baby out, but that elicited a strong rebuke from her physician.

"He told me very brusquely, 'If you continue to push, you are going to tear yourself up one side and down the other,' "Rose recalls. He scared us so bad. I did tear during the delivery and the doctor mumbled while he stitched me for an hour and fifteen minutes. The childbirth was very sobering, very traumatic. Afterward, I was extremely sore."

Rose could not sleep in the hospital, a phenomenon she attributed to her excitement and pain, and her desire to breastfeed her son. Even when Donald brought headphones and tapes of relaxing music to her in the hospital, she was unable to sleep. She stayed in the hospital an extra day because she had lost a great deal of blood during the birth. But by the time she left the hospital, Rose suspected things weren't quite right.

At home, Rose was still unable to sleep. During a home visit from a nurse practitioner, Rose told the nurse that she was angry at how her doctor had responded during the birth. She complained of her inability to sleep. The nurse reassured Rose that her feelings were normal. But the inability to sleep was a first clue. Within a week, Rose became psychotic.

"I started getting really intolerant of things. If the gardener came, the noise bothered me. I just couldn't stand it. I was also frustrated that I couldn't sleep. Then I began having thoughts, really clear thoughts, that someone had to die — be it me, the baby, my husband, my mother, or my father. I felt like I was losing my judgment. I knew I wasn't myself. That night I woke up my husband and told him everyone was going to die at midnight. This inability to know what was real and what wasn't was so frightening."

Rose was admitted to a psychiatric hospital but was released after a day and was told she could stop taking the tranquilizer she was given in the hospital so that she could resume breastfeeding. Without the medication, Rose relapsed into another, more severe, psychosis, imagining that she was having another baby. Again, an emergency room doctor prescribed medication and sent her home.

Rose's family and friends were shocked by her symptoms and were eager to help. Rose's coworkers went to a medical library and found information on postpartum psychosis. Rose's husband then searched and found the phone number for Postpartum Support International (PSI), a support society for women with postpartum depression and their families based in Santa Barbara, California. PSI members gave Donald information and support and referred him to a nearby specialist who treated postpartum psychosis. Donald called the specialist and Rose was quickly admitted to the psychiatric unit of the hospital where the doctor practiced. She was diagnosed with postpartum psychosis. Within a week, Rose began to recover.

But Rose's therapy was complicated. Nine years earlier, she had been raped at knifepoint in her home. During her recovery, Rose and her psychiatrist explored the many factors that seemed to contribute to Rose's psychosis and depression: perhaps a hormonal imbalance from childbirth; Post-Traumatic Stress Syndrome from the rape; and finally, a family history of depression. Rose's sister had suffered a postpartum psychosis after the birth of her third child and had been hospitalized. Rose's mother had also experienced depression.

Six weeks after Rose was released from the hospital, she had her first menstrual period since the birth of her son. That event triggered a relapse.

"I began having terrible thoughts, suicidal thoughts, thoughts about the rape. I was so afraid of every little noise. I was afraid that someone was going to break into the house."

Rose was hospitalized again. Again, she was so ill she had trouble distinguishing reality from fantasy. When Donald brought the baby to the hospital,

Rose rejected him and began having thoughts of wanting to hurt the baby. Rose gradually recovered from the psychosis but suffered from severe depression that doctors had difficulty treating. Finally, in addition to medication and counseling, her doctors tried an unusual treatment called sleep deprivation, waking Rose up each day at 3 A.M. in order to influence the production of mood-altering chemicals in the brain. Gradually, she began to recover from the depression. After a three-week hospitalization, Rose went home. She has battled relapses of depression and continues with therapy and maintenance doses of medications. In therapy, Rose has tried hard to overcome her tendency to blame her illness on her mothering abilities. She has fought to overcome her guilt that she was unable to care for her infant for many months after his birth. She has chosen a part-time career now instead of returning to her job full-time, as she had hoped to do. But Rose now recognizes and accepts that she was at high risk for postpartum illness and cannot blame herself. In addition to the possible influence of hormones in her postpartum illness, Rose had to battle a likely hereditary vulnerability to depression and the memories of her rape.

Victimization can include childhood sexual or physical abuse, marital or acquaintance rape, battering, sexual harassment in the workplace, and sexual abuse by a therapist or health care provider. Statistics show that victimization is so common that it should be considered in virtually all cases of depression in women.

Victims of abuse have many of the symptoms of persons with depression: hopelessness, helplessness, negative self-esteem, high levels of self-criticism, self-defeating attitudes and actions, and difficulties in relationships.

Studies have found that rates of sexual and physical abuse are higher than suspected and that victimization is a major factor in depression. One study estimated that 37 percent of women have had a significant experience of physical or sexual abuse before age twenty-one.[14] Some experts feel the numbers are even higher.

Since a large percentage of trauma is inflicted by a person known to the woman, perhaps trusted by or intimate with the woman, this type of victimization can erode a woman's faith in her ability to maintain healthy relationships, a key aspect to her psychological health. Women who are verbally, physically, or sexually abused in childhood often compensate with personality styles that are highly controlling. But having a baby can shatter this self-control and allow buried anxieties from childhood to emerge.

"Many of these women are overachievers," says Dr. Deborah Sichel. "They strive to achieve. They strive to be perfect. This character trait really is established for them, and then it really doesn't work once they have a baby."

Uncovering a past history of victimization can be difficult for the health care provider, however. You may have been reluctant to tell your doctor, for example, or may have minimized the details or glossed over the experience, particularly if you were abused by a family member. This is common. Historically, women who said they were sexually or physically abused in childhood have been disbelieved or blamed by mental health professionals. In addition, some women do not recall incidents of victimization that occurred in childhood until they are in therapy.

Since having a baby commonly brings back memories of childhood, this may be the time when childhood abuse is recalled. If you are a survivor of abuse, don't downplay the significance of this experience as a factor in your postpartum depression. However painful, you should deal with the abuse as part of your total recovery. This situation needs professional guidance. Find a counselor or therapist who can help you with both past and current concerns. Take heart. You will emerge from the postpartum illness much more at peace with yourself. (For ongoing support, see the Resources section for groups that assist those recovering from abuse.)

If you are presently in an abusive relationship or environment, help is available. In a 1992 report in the prestigious *Journal of the American Medical Association* (*JAMA*), experts urged all physicians to specifically look for and ask women about any possible history of victimization. Sadly, a number of women are first battered when they become pregnant, the study notes. Physicians should be on alert to provide battered women with a full range of services and advocacy, including emergency shelter, legal and medical care, court accompaniment, and referrals to counseling support groups. If you are presently in an abusive environment, talk to your physician about help in this manner. If necessary, ask your physician to refer to the May 5, 1992, *JAMA*.

CHAPTER SIX

Hormones: Powerful Regulators of Mood

W omen who are treated for postpartum psychiatric disorders are usually told that their illnesses result from chemicals in their bodies that are out of sync. Even women with postpartum blues usually link their tearfulness and exhaustion to the catchall explanation: Hormones.

In the previous chapters, we saw how several factors can lead to postpartum illness. But for many women, hormones are probably the underlying cause or major contributing factor to the illness. In other words, postpartum depression is a biological illness with psychiatric symptoms.

The hormonal-cause theory of postpartum illness is controversial for several reasons, however. One is that it has yet to be completely proven. The second is that the psychological and lifestyle factors discussed earlier are known to be very significant in the development of the illness. Finally, some health professionals — and some women — are reluctant to blame anything on hormones because this explanation implies that women are powerless over their bodies.

"Postpartum psychosis is controversial for the same reason PMS [premenstrual syndrome] is. Some say it's a sexist thing to say women are not in control of their minds but are affected by their hormones," says Dr. Robert Sadoff, a professor of psychiatry at the University of Pennsylvania School of medicine.

Despite the absence of proof that hormones trigger postpartum psychiatric illness, there is ample reason to believe that hormones contribute heavily to the disorders. A simple overview of what happens to the body during and after pregnancy reveals just how powerful hormones are.

Understanding the Role of Hormones

Hormones are chemicals that determine our body size, temperament, and activity level. They are part of the body's endocrine system and are produced by endocrine glands. Hormones are transported by body fluids, such as blood, to specific organs and tissues to influence their functioning. If the hormone level changes, so does the functioning of the organ. The hormones act like chemical messengers that travel through the bloodstream to special receptors in the body that are designed specifically to receive them.

To understand how postpartum illness is triggered by hormones, we need to look at the role of the hormones produced by the pituitary, adrenal, and thyroid glands. The pituitary gland is located deep inside the head, behind the nose. It is called the body's master gland because it produces many of the hormones that control other glands. The pituitary is divided in two parts: the foremost part, or anterior lobe, and the back, or posterior lobe.

The hormones produced in the anterior lobe stimulate other glands or organs into action, such as the gonadotropin hormones that stimulate the ovary to release an egg each month. And, most important for understanding postpartum psychiatric illness, the anterior lobe stimulates the production of ACTH (adrenal-cortex-stimulating hormone) and TSH (thyroid-stimulating hormone).

The thyroid gland is a butterfly-shaped gland in the neck just below the larynx. Thyroid-stimulating hormone (TSH) stimulates the thyroid gland to produce its own hormones.

The pituitary secretes spurts of ACTH throughout the day, which then stimulates the adrenal glands to produce hormones.

(These spurts are more frequent during predawn hours and become less frequent throughout the day. This is why we suffer from changes in our biological clocks — with jet lag, for example.) The adrenals are triangular-shaped glands atop the kidneys. The adrenal produces a group of hormones referred to as steroids. This includes the glucocorticoids, which help regulate the metabolism of glucose (blood sugar) and other nutrients. The adrenals also trigger production of the sex hormones androgen and estrogen. Estrogen is the chemical that activates the ovaries to release an egg every month. Progesterone is released in the second half of the monthly cycle, causing the uterine lining to thicken and prepare for pregnancy. If an egg is not fertilized, the progesterone stops secreting and the lining is lost in menstruation.

Cortisol is the most abundant glucocorticoid in humans. Corticosteroid secretion is the particular hormone thought to be linked to our biological or internal clocks. The liver can metabolize cortisol into cortisone, a steroid that is used to treat allergic disorders like asthma or inflammations such as arthritis. The side effects of cortisone, however, can include euphoria, alertness, and insomnia. And when cortisone is administered and then withdrawn, additional psychiatric symptoms are sometimes observed.

What Happens During Pregnancy

During pregnancy the thyroid enlarges somewhat and increases its production of a chemical called thyroxine. This raises the body's metabolic rate to provide the energy needed for the developing fetus and the chemical changes taking place in a woman's body.

The adrenal glands also produce more hormones during pregnancy. And the placenta becomes a "hormone factory," turning out large quantities of estrogen, progesterone, ACTH, and special pregnancy hormones to nourish the fetus.

The mystery of what causes postpartum psychiatric illness really begins during the last three months of pregnancy when estrogen and progesterone rise to the highest levels a woman will ever experience. But, when the placenta is delivered, usually within thirty minutes of birth, the levels of these hormones in the blood plunge to nearly zero within twenty-four hours. It is this rapid transformation that is now the center of one avenue of research on postpartum psychiatric illness. So dramatic is this shift in hormones that one expert described a woman's hormonal state after childbirth as "comparable to that following menopause."[1]

Physicians have long recognized that the loss of the placenta and its hormones can cause dizziness, sweating, and heart palpitations. But what the sudden, drastic loss of these hormones does to a woman's psychiatric health is far less understood.

HAMILTON'S THEORY

Dr. James Hamilton was among the first experts to suggest that a chemical imbalance can trigger psychiatric symptoms after childbirth. He wrote of this explanation in his 1962 book *Postpartum Psychiatric Problems.*

According to Hamilton, as the placenta develops, it produces estrogen and progesterone. The levels of estrogen and progesterone peak before delivery to the order of ten times the maximum women experience when they are not pregnant. The production of progesterone may be twenty-five times higher than in the nonpregnant state. After delivery of the baby, the levels drop and remain low until the menstrual cycle resumes, usually about six weeks later. Also during pregnancy the thyroid and anterior pituitary glands enlarge. And experts suggest that the enlarged pituitary produces an increased amount of several hormones, including the TSH. The adrenal cortex is the final parameter in Hamilton's theory (in addition to estrogen and progesterone, and thyroid hormones).

Here is how he believes the hormonal imbalance occurs: In the last weeks of pregnancy, the metabolism speeds up because of enormous quantities of estrogen and progesterone. The pituitary gland responds by handling increased blood circulation. The pituitary sends hormones ACTH and TSH to the other glands of the body to stimulate the production of their hormones. At delivery, estrogen and progesterone fall. In addition, the pituitary hormones fall, especially ACTH and TSH. "With the foot off the accelerator, the circulation and apparent cellular activity of the pituitary decrease very rapidly. Its blood supply drops within hours after delivery," Hamilton says.

The fall in the ACTH causes a drop in substances called cortisol and free cortisol. And, if the drop is too deep, the phenomenon of psychosis occurs. (Some experts suggest that the drop in cortisol creates a postpartum psychosis with a sudden, early onset. And the changes in thyroxin result in a syndrome more like major postpartum depression. In general, more medical experts tend to believe that a hormonal imbalance is responsible for sudden psychosis, and fewer experts support the theory that hormonal imbalances cause postpartum depression that begins weeks after childbirth.)

"These disorders are organic disorders, with important but secondary psychological complications," Hamilton argues. "They are probably disorders of simple hormonal deficit. They are disorders which we should be able to treat as specific and identified deficits, and prevent by interrupting the sequence of hormonal events which leads to the deficits." But, he adds, "We have not distinguished ourselves in pursuing these rather obvious clues."

SOME EVIDENCE

The fact is, there is no direct proof to support this theory. But experts point to several pieces of evidence that indicate the theory should be pursued in much more detail. For example, findings from a 1983 study showed that estrogen and progesterone levels were lower among women with the blues than those without the blues.[2] Another study found that the greater the progesterone drop from before delivery to after, the more likely women were to rate themselves as depressed. The lower the estrogen level, the more likely sleep disturbances were seen.[3] In addition, some experiments in which women have been given supplements of hormones to offset the drastic drop of hormones after delivery appear to have been successful.[4]

NOT ENOUGH PROOF

Still, additional research is sorely needed to understand the possible effects of hormones during pregnancy and delivery on postpartum psychiatric illness. According to Dr. Robert B. Filer in *Postpartum Psychiatric Illness*, "The association between the endocrine changes after delivery and postpartum depression has never been well established. Although it would be rewarding to be able to isolate an endocrine cause for the depression, no such association has been delineated to date. All reports of the correlation between postpartum depression and hormonal changes have been anecdotal and not the result of prospective controlled studies." Filer argues that the desire to find a medical cause for the disorder "has led to several attempts at treatment, none of which have demonstrated a direct association between the medication and the results."

That is not to say that, with more research, an explanation for the dramatic rise in mood disorders in postpartum women won't be identified. According to Dr. Lee S. Cohen, an expert in reproductive psychiatry at Massachusetts General Hospital and Harvard Medical School, "Our recent review of the literature suggests there is no good data consistently supporting a single neurochemical dysregulator in patients who suffer from postpartum depression, whether you look at estrogen, progesterone, prolactin, or oxytocin. It is my hope that we will develop neuroendocrine probes that will be better predictors and will speak better to the physiology of puerperal illness."

WHY IT'S SO DIFFICULT TO STUDY HORMONES

Why can't we measure a woman's hormones during pregnancy and afterward and compare the levels? Why can't the hormone levels of the woman with postpartum depression then be compared with that of women without depression? These are the million-dollar questions, according to postpartum expert Ricardo Fernandez.

There are several reasons why this simple suggestion doesn't work in theory. One reason it's difficult to compare hormone levels is because of individual variability. For example, some women may be particularly vulnerable to depression when their estrogen or progesterone levels drop to a certain level while other women with similar hormone levels will be unaffected.

There is simply no particular level that predicts psychiatric symptoms, Fernandez explains. Rather, it is the relative change in levels from the pregnant to the nonpregnant state that is probably causing the symptoms. "You can test hormones by just getting a blood sample, that's no problem. The problem is that, let's say the normal range for progesterone is 450 to 2,500 units. Let's say you take 10 moms during pregnancy and two months postpartum and they're all symptomatic. Some will come in with a progesterone of 450, another will be 1,800, another will be 200. There is no correlation between symptoms and progesterone levels. The symptoms are probably related not necessarily to the level, but rather to the drop in the hormones that occurs in the postpartum period. There's no real way to measure that. Even if we could measure it, we don't know what that slope is, so we wouldn't be able to tell what the normal rate is."

Hormone levels change abruptly and unpredictably, he adds. It is very difficult to test a woman's hormone levels on one day and link it to particular moods or behaviors. "After the mom delivers and until she gets her first period, her hormone levels are all over the place," he says. "Progesterone might be doing one thing, estrogen another, and thyroid another. I don't know when someone is having symptoms whether it's the progesterone, estrogen, or thyroid. The only thing that has been documented in terms of thyroid function is that it's high at delivery, it drops after childbirth, and goes under normal between two and five months and some women become symptomatic in their depression at that point. Then the majority of women, slowly over the course of time [about a year], become normal again in terms of their thyroid function."

THE POSTPARTUM THYROID PROBLEM

In fact, the good news about postpartum psychiatric illness is that at least one group of hormones and their functions — the thyroid hormones — are relatively well understood. The problem is that thyroid imbalances in new mothers are often overlooked by physicians.

Thyroid levels play a significant role in mental illness, especially among women. Because the thyroid hormones are essential to the body's metabolism, failure of the thyroid can affect all the organs and hormonal systems in the body. There are two general types of thyroid disorders: too much thyroid production, called hyperthyroidism, and too little thyroid production, called hypothyroidism. Hyperthyroidism causes an acceleration of the body's metabolism; a person will find it hard to rest, will feel nervous and shaky, and may lose weight. Hypothyroidism causes sleepiness, weight gain, lethargy, fatigue, swelling, and dry skin and hair. Women will notice that their periods are heavy and more frequent.

Hypothyroidism is associated not only with slowed mental processes but with significant depressive effect. Symptoms of subclinical hypothyroidism are agitated depression, some physical symptoms such as loss of hair, menstrual changes, skin changes, edema, marked irritability, and premenstrual worsening. Women with postpartum thyroid show impaired concentration, impaired memory, and difficulty in performing work.

Studies show imbalances in thyroid production are common in women after they have babies. Up to 9 percent of all obstetrics patients develop thyroid dysfunction in the postpartum period. Most of these cases of thyroiditis are temporary and may even correct themselves. Others require medical treatment. But despite its common occurrence and simple steps required to detect and treat thyroid disorders, they are often overlooked in postpartum women.[5] However, all women complaining of fatigue or mood disorders in the postpartum period should be examined for thyroid disorder.

Postpartum thyroid disease usually occurs from two to five months postpartum but can occur anytime in the first six months. More frequent assessment of the psychiatric status of women in the six months of the postpartum period would probably turn up more depression associated with thyroid dysfunction, experts say.

Why is thyroid disorder so prevalent after a woman has a baby? The answer to this question isn't entirely known. But, in the postpartum period, thyroid disorder is considered an autoimmune disease precipitated by postpartum changes in the immune system. That is, the stress of pregnancy and delivering a baby may trigger the disorder. For example, it's well recognized that other autoimmune diseases such as myasthenia gravis and rheumatoid arthritis may go away during pregnancy but flare up in the postpartum period.

Any woman with a history of thyroid disease or who has a first-degree relative with it should have thyroid tests done in the first trimester of pregnancy. If a problem is evident, she should be monitored throughout pregnancy and into the postpartum period.

Many cases of postpartum thyroid disorder correct themselves over time without treatment. But studies show that about 3.5 percent of patients with postpartum thyroiditis remain permanently hypothyroid. And women with postpartum thyroid disorder have a 10 to 25 percent chance of thyroiditis in subsequent pregnancies.[6]

OTHER QUESTIONS: PREMENSTRUAL SYNDROME AND BREASTFEEDING

There are many other questions, clues, theories, and observations about the effects of hormones on mood during and after pregnancy. Two of the most interesting questions involve the link between premenstrual syndrome (PMS) and postpartum disorders and the role breastfeeding plays in postpartum disorders.

The fact that women are least likely to become depressed during pregnancy and most likely after pregnancy suggests the role of hormones on mood. But many women report they feel euphoric during pregnancy. According to Barbara Parry, a psychiatrist at the University of California–San Diego, this raises the question of whether there is a physiological mechanism during pregnancy that protects a woman from depression. In her extensive research, Parry has noted that euphoria is common during the late follicular phase of the menstrual cycle when estrogen levels are increasing. Further, depression often occurs in the late luteal (premenstrual phase) of the cycle when hormone levels are declining. This euphoria-to-depression cycle mirrors what can happen to some women from pregnancy to the postpartum period.

During pregnancy and the late follicular phase of the menstrual cycle, hormone levels increase and mood is often high. But during the postpartum period and the premenstrual phase of the cycle, hormones decline and a woman is more vulnerable to sadness.

Many women have mild or severe mood changes premenstrually. About 5 percent have severe PMS including symptoms of depressed mood; irritability; hostility; anxiety; changes in sleep, appetite, and energy; and somatic symptoms. It is common for women with postpartum mood disorders to report having suffered from PMS.

No one knows whether the same type of hormones or hormonal fluctuations might affect women premenstrually and in the postpartum period. But Katharina Dalton has advocated the use of progesterone premenstrually because she believes PMS is caused by a progesterone deficiency. She has also used progesterone in the postpartum period. Her studies — both in the premenstrual period and in the postpartum period — claim to show mood improvement in women who receive progesterone. But other studies have not shown a link between progesterone and improved mood. And, blood tests show some women with severe PMS have normal progesterone levels.

Meanwhile, Parry suggests that the reproductive hormones could affect mood directly or indirectly by their effect on the neurotransmitter or circadian systems. Both these systems are linked to depressive illness.

The biological clock is also called our circadian rhythms. According to Parry, estrogen and progesterone can alter the synthesis, release, uptake, and degradation of brain chemicals (neurotransmitters) that are so important to mood, such as norepinephrine, dopamine, and serotonin. The gonadal steroids also affect the thyroid, cortisol, prolactin, and opiate hormonal mechanisms; and these hormones, too, influence neurotransmitters.

According to a theory developed by Parry, the gonadal steroids affect biological clock mechanisms that are connected to mood. Parry suggests that when the ovarian hormones decline — as in the premenstrual and postpartum periods — they may upset and destabilize the neurotransmitter, neuroendocrine, and biological clock mechanisms. This chain reaction, she suggests, may set the stage for mood disorders.

In a recent study, Parry found that patients with PMS secrete lower amounts of a brain chemical commonly released at night, which is evidence that biological clocks or circadian rhythms might contribute to the syndrome. The chemical is melatonin. She speculates that perhaps other forms of depression, such as postpartum illness, are linked to a desynchronization of the body's biological clocks. "The theory for depressive patients is that when these clocks get out of sync with each other, certain people may be prone to mood disorders," she says.

Other studies have shown that estrogen and progesterone are among the few known internal modulators of circadian clocks. Thus, according to Parry, among PMS patients, changes in sensitivity to these reproductive hormones during the menstrual cycle may desynchronize body clocks.

The same thing might happen due to hormonal changes in the postpartum period. But much more research is required to understand what similarities may exist between PMS and postpartum mood disorders and what can be learned from the treatment of each.

Some evidence exists for the link between estrogen, serotonin, and mood. In animal studies, British researchers showed that estrogen helps the brain use more serotonin by creating more receptors for serotonin, which are sites in the brain for the chemical to be absorbed. Serotonin, as you recall, is the brain neurotransmitter that is so important to mood and sleep. Although researchers have known that fact for some time, the British research is the first to show how estrogen provides an important link.[7] This evidence may eventually help explain why women generally suffer depression far more frequently than men (see Table 6-1). Estrogen levels in women drop prior to menstruation, after childbirth, and at menopause.

Table 6-1. *Women Suffer from Depression More Than Men*

Age	Depression in previous year		Depression at any time in life	
	Women (%)	*Men (%)*	*Women (%)*	*Men(%)*
18-29	5.8	3.1	11.0	6.4
30-44	7.9	2.7	15.0	6.6
45-64	3.6	1.7	9.3	3.6
65 and older	1.5	0.6	3.3	1.6

Source: Columbia University, The Commonwealth Fund Commission on Women's Health, March, 1995.

Although estrogen and progesterone are considered the key hormones that might affect mood in the postpartum period, some researchers are exploring the role of prolactin, the hormone that establishes breast milk, in causing mood disturbances. Until recently, little attention has been paid to the roles of breastfeeding and weaning in postpartum psychiatric disorders, say researchers Virginia L. Susman of Cornell University and her colleague Jack L. Katz. Significant hormonal changes occur during the process of weaning. Susman and Katz have identified several cases in which weaning an infant from breastfeeding has been an apparent trigger in postpartum psychiatric illness.[8] Other studies have shown that elevated levels of prolactin make women prone to depression.

NEUROTRANSMITTERS

Scientists have also begun to question the effects of estrogen and progesterone on the chemicals in the brain that are known to effect mood and psychological functioning. These brain chemicals are called neurotransmitters.

Neurotransmitters are chemical messengers that carry electro-chemical signals between nerve cells. They are concentrated in areas of the brain that control drives for sex, hunger, and thirst. A particular class of neurotransmitters are called biogenic amines. Imbalances created by too much or too little of these biogenic amines — serotonin, norepinephrine, and dopamine — are thought to be at the root of biochemical depression.

Serotonin, which is involved in all aspects of human behavior, interacts with other biochemicals involved in the regulation of the neuroendocrine system, which controls the thyroid, adrenal glands, and ovaries. Thus, a deficiency of serotonin, which appears to occur frequently in depression, would affect all these other systems. The lack of serotonin is thought to cause emotionally volatile and impulsive behaviors.

Thus, the workings of the pituitary gland, thyroid, and adrenals; the levels of estrogen and progesterone; and the functioning of the neurotransmitter serotonin and perhaps others are all pieces of the puzzle. To varying degrees, these factors most likely play a role in the majority of postpartum psychiatric illnesses.

Obsessive-Compulsive Disorder

In studying women with obsessive-compulsive disorder (OCD) in the postpartum period, Deborah Sichel of Harvard Medical School has suggested that hormone fluctuations may affect neurotransmitters producing the common symptom of anxiety. Anxiety is a significant symptom throughout the range of postpartum disorders. "Perhaps the one common symptom that all these psychiatric syndromes seem to have that occur after giving birth appears to be an anxiety response. We're starting to look very carefully at what that is and what does it mean in terms of inferring certain features."

Anxiety during pregnancy can be a predictor for postpartum illness, Sichel notes. "This is anxiety that is not related to the normal fears of mothers just worrying 'Is my baby going to be OK? Am I gaining enough weight?' These are normal kinds of concerns. This is an anxiety that really develops above that and does not seem related in any way to any particular stimulant that is going on."

In a study of twenty patients with obsessive-compulsive disorder in the postpartum period, Sichel found the women commonly have anxious, obsessive thoughts about harming the baby, depression, hopelessness, and loss of sleep. "All come in undiagnosed, feeling ashamed and terrified about what is going on," she says. "Their first thoughts seem to be, 'Well, I could drown this baby' or feeling as if they could drown this baby. There is not a voice. This is not a psychotic symptom. These people are absolutely in contact with reality."

The obsessive thoughts — often involving knives, scissors, or anything that can hurt the baby — can become persistent. "So people start to move away from any kind of activity interacting with any device with which they could harm the babies . . . . These women want these babies. They care about the babies. They love the babies. And their thoughts are intrusive. They all develop avoidant types of behaviors to cope with these thoughts. You don't have to be any kind of a child-development expert to know what an impact this must have on the mother-infant relationship."

The women are often reluctant to admit their thoughts or ask for help. She adds: "These women are terrified because they have no control over this thought process." But, in most of these cases, it's unlikely that the mother will harm the baby.

What does this mean? According to Sichel, studies show OCD involves the release of a neurotransmitter — a chemical messenger — between nerve cells. But there is a problem in the uptake of the message to the next nerve terminal; in particular, in nerve cells designed to absorb the neurotransmitter serotonin. OCD is relatively common, affecting between 2 and 3 percent of the population. It is often treated successfully with serotonergic re-uptake drugs like Prozac and Anafranil.

What is interesting is that studies show that the withdrawal of estrogen can affect serotonergic receptors. At birth, in just twenty-four hours, estrogen drops from the highest levels of a woman's life to its lowest. So this estrogen plunge may be a mechanism to trigger OCD or a similar syndrome such as postpartum depression with anxiety.

But, since OCD doesn't affect all women, there may also be some underlying biological weakness, Sichel says. Her studies raise the question of whether giving a woman estrogen supplements after birth might prevent postpartum disorder.

Much of the research on hormonal underpinnings of postpartum illness is new and ever changing. This is a major reason why women encounter such a wide range of reactions and treatment options when they seek help for postpartum illness. The good news is that, even though the causes of these disorders are not completely understood, a number of treatment options have been shown to work.

CHAPTER SEVEN

The Many Options for Treatment

During the difficult days of a postpartum illness, you may wonder if you will ever experience the delight of caring for and loving your baby. You may question whether you will ever revel in the joy of parenthood — whether you will ever fall asleep at night, warmly and pleasantly exhausted, and give thanks to God for your glorious children and happy life. For almost all women with postpartum illness, the answer is yes, you will. Postpartum disorders are highly treatable.

If you have a more mild illness — such as maternity blues or mild postpartum depression — the symptoms will often vanish spontaneously after a few days or weeks. For women with more serious illness — including acute psychosis — there are a number of good treatments that are often used concurrently to produce a full recovery. Even women with more serious illnesses often recover on their own, without treatment. But the possibility of long-lasting depression or recurrent depressions later makes it imperative for women with more serious illnesses to seek treatment.

"The earlier the symptoms are recognized and treated, the better the outcome," says psychiatrist Barbara Parry, an expert on women's mood disorders at the University of California–San Diego. But, too often, she says, a woman who seems to feel distant from her child is not taken seriously when that may be an early clue to an impending psychosis. If psychosis isn't treated promptly, she notes, startling behavior, such as paranoid delusions, may set in and then the illness becomes very difficult to treat. "Without aggressive management and early detection, the symptoms may extend into the second and third year postpartum." Conversely, if the symptoms of psychosis are treated early, they may be resolved within a single week.

One of the myths that has developed around postpartum illness is that it is more difficult to treat than other nonpregnancy-related mood disorders. This is probably not true, experts say. But the inability of women to seek prompt treatment — and the failure of health professionals in spotting postpartum illness — may delay treatment in a great many women. And the longer the illness goes on untreated, the more difficult it may be to reach full recovery.

What kind of treatment is effective for postpartum illnesses? There is no clear-cut answer to that question, notes Parry. "Because these illnesses can be so devastating to the individual and her family, treatment approaches have utilized whatever interventions have been immediately useful and available."

In general, treatment for postpartum illness involves psychotherapy and/or medication. Psychotherapy, including family therapy, is usually a must for postpartum patients. Pharmacotherapy, or drug therapy, is also common for moderate and severe depression as well as psychosis, obsessive-compulsive disorder, and anxiety disorder related to the postpartum period. Phototherapy and electroconvulsive therapy are other treatment options that are seldom used, for reasons that are discussed later.

Whatever you do, it's important for you, your physicians and therapists, and your family to discuss all the options and agree on the course of treatment. Remember that the choice of treatment depends on the nature and severity of the depressive symptoms. Treatment should be individualized to meet the circumstances of each particular woman. "There is no absolute standard of care. Each woman that I encounter is evaluated according to her very,

very specific needs," says one of the nation's most experienced authorities on postpartum illness, Dr. Deborah Sichel.

The irony of postpartum illness is that, despite the lack of understanding about what causes the disorder and lack of research regarding treatments specific to the postpartum period, many treatments have proven successful. But, this dearth of research should serve as a reminder that you and your health practitioners need to remain open-minded about therapy and poised to try something new. What may work for one woman may not work for the next.

"You can't just say 'A equals B.' We're working with each one woman as her own biochemical, spiritual, physical self. And you can't say, what works for Sally works for Mary," says Jeanne Watson Driscoll, a psychotherapist in private practice in Massachusetts.

Most postpartum experts agree, however, that women benefit most from a team approach to treatment. Each member of the team — nurses, social workers, occupational therapists, psychologists, and psychiatrists — can address the specific needs of you and your family. Postpartum illness is a complex disorder affecting numerous aspects of your life — your physical health, feelings, and relationships. A good approach to treatment will include psychotherapy, counseling, family meetings, and discharge planning, perhaps along with drug therapy, such as hormones, thyroid supplements, antidepressants, or antianxiety medications.

You might be treated in a health maintenance organization, a community mental health center, a hospital department of psychiatry or outpatient psychiatric clinic, a university or medical school affiliated program, a state hospital outpatient clinic, a family service/ social agency, or a private clinic. Your health professional may be a family doctor, obstetrician-gynecologist, psychiatrist, psychologist, social worker, or marriage and family therapist. What is really important is not where the help is coming from but how knowledgeable the caregivers are regarding your postpartum illness. The biggest problem with treatment of postpartum disorders is that too many health professionals are uninformed about the illness. This results in women being mistreated — sometimes for months and by several different practitioners — before they finally fall into the "right" hands and receive appropriate care. The story of Beth is a tragic example.

> *Beth was twenty-five years old when she gave birth to her son. She was a cheerful person who loved children. And, after five years of marriage, she looked forward to having her own. But Beth's personality changed abruptly just a few days after the birth. She became quiet and within a few days was worrying over irrational things. She plunged into a depression and, one week after childbirth, tried to suffocate herself with a pillow. She was hospitalized and began several months of various treatments including antidepressants, psychotherapy, lithium, and electroconvulsive therapy. But Beth, her husband, and her parents were not lucky enough to find the right health professional who could provide successful treatment. The mishandling of her care began with her obstetrician, who downplayed her initial symptoms of distress. Another doctor rejected Beth by telling her, over the phone, that he couldn't help her. One of the first psychiatrists to treat her failed to see that she was suicidal. Beth received very few of the diagnostic tests that are so crucial to an accurate diagnosis, such as the thyroid tests that are commonly ordered for postpartum patients.*
> *The hospitalizations were nightmares for Beth and her family. Beth was verbally abused in a highly regarded psychiatric hospital. One day, recalls Beth's mother, the nurses on the ward refused to let Beth see her baby because she had not gotten up in time and followed her schedule for the day. But,*

Beth's parents contend, their daughter was so delusional and confused that she couldn't even comprehend a television program, let alone follow an orderly schedule. In another incident, a psychologist humiliated Beth by demanding that she tell her family all the problems she thought she was causing them. At another point, Beth's doctors surmised that she feared her baby and decided to put the baby in the hospital with her. Beth did fear hurting the baby. And she became progressively worse as the care of the baby was forced on her.

"They never picked up on Beth's fear of herself. They always attributed it to the fear of the baby, fear of handling the baby. I knew that wasn't true," Beth's mother recalled. "She hadn't been with the baby for two months and suddenly she was thrown with the baby for an entire day, not knowing the baby's schedule or anything . . . They treated Beth like she was stupid. She got so she wouldn't talk to anyone on the floor because of the punishments she got. She was treated as though this was an ordinary depression; that postpartum had nothing to do with it."

Beth's medications were changed too frequently for the full effects to become noticeable. Her electroconvulsive therapy was cut short after four treatments, again too early to produce results. Physicians never gave Beth's parents a reason for terminating the treatment early.

Eventually, Beth left the hospital, still ill, and later committed suicide. A few years later, however, at a meeting of people interested in postpartum illness, Beth's mother addressed women with postpartum illness and the professionals who treat them: "Don't give up. There is nothing that can't be solved somehow."

This story is troubling and, fortunately, incidents like this one are rare. But it serves a useful purpose here to illustrate how imperative it is for families to seek treatment from an expert on postpartum illness. Be suspicious of a practitioner who seems to judge you or tries to invalidate your feelings. Some doctors simply won't listen to you or make a sincere attempt to understand. Unknowledgeable doctors sometimes label women neurotic, psychotic, or schizophrenic, or tell them they have general depression unrelated to childbirth.

It is crucial that the health practitioner treats you within the context of the postpartum period, says Seattle therapist and postpartum expert Dawn Gruen, who has written and lectured on the disorder. Psychotherapists and psychiatrists should be trained in the issues of the postpartum period. Untrained practitioners may tell you there is no such thing as postpartum depression or may spend time discussing some tangential issue, such as your father's alcoholism.

"You have to address the issues in the context of the postpartum time," Gruen says. "It's the uniqueness of this time that makes working with these women very different from other kinds of life stages."

In its report on women and depression, experts from the American Psychological Association (APA) stressed that therapists must be knowledgeable about the psychology of women and gender differences related to the cause and treatment of depression. They must be empathetic to women's special needs and understand women's different modes of expressing depression. There are three issues that deserve special attention regarding women and depression: menstrual cycle effects, co-occurrence of symptoms that are linked to past victimization, and hormonal factors. Depression among women tends to be linked with many gender-related biological, psychological, and social factors including reproductive events; personality factors related to competence and self-esteem; coping styles such as learned helplessness; physical and sexual abuse; and discrimination and poverty, the APA report noted.

"Psychopharmacologists and other therapists must not attempt to provide treatment to female depressed patients unless they are adequately trained in victimization theory and clinical practice; without such training, the risks for inadequate treatment are too great, especially for women with complicated depression," the APA task force reported.[1] It is impossible to know how many mental health professionals fit that criteria. But given the lack of attention and research to women's mental health problems, it would not be unreasonable to suspect that the majority do not. Despite decades of increased awareness regarding women's issues, most psychologists in a national survey had never taken a single course on the special problems women face, according to a 1990 study. "They had taken no courses that focus on such obvious female concerns as rape, incest, battering, abortion, and menopause," said psychologist Laurie Mintz of the University of Southern California.[2]

Psychiatrists are equally at fault for failing to distinguish women's unique problems. Moreover, only about 40 percent of the nation's psychiatrists are women. "In general, psychiatrists are not knowledgeable about what it means to be at home and to take care of small children," says social worker and postpartum expert Penny Handford, a Canadian who has studied the disorder.

Because of the complexity of women's mental health issues, the APA report suggested that women with depression consider the services of female therapists. "Some female therapists may have a special empathetic knowledge that may be very helpful in treatment of depression, by virtue of being female and sharing affective connectiveness with their women clients," the report said.

THE INITIAL ASSESSMENT

A woman with postpartum illness who is brought — for the first time — into an emergency room or doctor's office is usually in a crisis. She may have just suffered a panic attack or a bout of agitated mania. She may have mentioned suicide or tried to kill herself. She has usually been crying for days, has not slept well for weeks, has stopped eating, and can barely care for her child. Her husband is beside himself with confusion and concern. Her family feels shocked and helpless. The woman herself is distraught, confused, and blind with fatigue. She thinks she is going crazy. She cannot comprehend what bizarre force has taken over her life. She is wracked with guilt that she can neither appreciate nor care for her child. She wonders what in the world has happened to the person she used to be.

The health professional facing this woman and her horrified husband has much work to do. It's important that her immediate needs are met at the same time that health professionals are beginning the process of working toward a diagnosis and treatment plan.

Because postpartum illness can take on many different forms, depending on the woman and her unique circumstances, the professional must — first and foremost — make a careful, critical assessment of the case before him or her. Some women will downplay the symptoms by telling the doctor that they simply have "postpartum blues." But postpartum blues is usually over and gone by two weeks after childbirth. If a woman is still distressed at six, eight, ten weeks or later, "We should be screaming that it's not the blues," says Dr. Lee S. Cohen, expert in psychiatry at Massachusetts General Hospital and Harvard Medical School.

To do this, the practitioner must listen to the symptoms involved. Oftentimes, a family member can best relate what has happened to the woman, says Barbara Conley, a psychiatric social worker at the Pregnancy and Infant/Parent Center at Western Psychiatric Institute in Pittsburgh. Family members should be encouraged to attend the initial assessment. "Many times the women are so dysfunctional that they can't tell us a whole lot. So it's real important to have those family members there."

The immediate safety of the mother and her child must also be assessed, including a discussion on whether hospitalization is needed.

And, if it is not, on who is available to watch and care for the mother and children at home.

Finally, within the initial assessment, the practitioner needs to reassure this grieving couple that help is on the way. No health professional should ever doubt the mercy of those words. The woman and her family must be given hope.

"This is the time to tell women they're not going crazy, that it's alright to talk to other people, that they don't have to be afraid of their bizarre thoughts or their frightening thoughts, that it's a time when they can begin to understand someone else in the world has felt this," says Dawn Gruen. During this time, the health professional should, if possible, give the family a name for the illness — postpartum depression, maternity blues, postpartum psychosis — even if the clinicians have not yet determined the cause.

THE INITIAL PHASE OF TREATMENT

During the next few weeks, the acute phase of the illness shall be addressed. Shortly after the initial assessment — often at that very meeting — the professional should conduct a physical evaluation, including blood tests to look for any physical problems that could be causing the symptoms, such as thyroid disease or anemia.

The mother's physical history must be reviewed as soon as possible, including her reproductive history. Questions regarding the nature of past childbirth experiences and whether she has ever had premenstrual syndrome are crucial in helping the professional identify a postpartum disorder.

An often overlooked part of the assessment is inquiry into past substance abuse problems or past victimization. The failure to address past victimization may result in poorer results at psychotherapy and inappropriate reliance on medications, according to the APA task force on Women and Depression.

Within these first few days and weeks, the safety of the mother and child must be consistently reviewed. Family members must begin to be educated about the illness. A "safety net" must be con-structed for the mother and her children. "In order for any inter-ventions to work, these women must be supported all day long," said one therapist.[3]

To persuade the mother and her family to address the imme-diate issues at hand, therapists may ask her to set aside other issues, problems, and concerns for a short period of time. This is a period in which the family agrees to forego making any decisions about relationships, the home, work, and so forth, until this crisis has passed. This is especially important for couples who come in on the verge of separation or divorce.

At this point, the mother should begin learning about her dis-order and start to address her feelings, which may have been long denied or buried behind guilt and embarrassment. As a first step, Conley asks women to rate their feelings throughout the day. "Helping them to rate it is the beginning of getting control over the feeling. That helps them want to communicate it and evaluate it. When you go to evaluate something or someone you are begin-ning to have control over it."

Mothers are also encouraged to begin talking about the ways in which their expectations of childbirth and parenting have col-lided with the unexpected. After all, Conley notes, "This is hardly the experience they thought they were going to have."

You're being robbed of the most important moments of your life.

THE SECOND PHASE OF TREATMENT

The next phase of treatment typically lasts from about six weeks to four months and should focus on stabilization. In this period, eval-uating the safety of the mother and baby must continue.

By this time, drug treatment should be well under way with the necessary trial-and-error period completed. It often takes several weeks for antidepressants to reach their full effect, and evaluation of their usefulness must wait until then. Women who are not experiencing significant recovery from drug therapy by this time should be presented with alternative therapy choices, such as different medications or perhaps even a change in doctors or therapists.

A woman may also need to begin addressing her feelings about the illness and the loss of interactive time with her infant. Care of the baby by friends and relatives can be gradually reduced as she is able to take on more child care duties. She can begin to re-establish her bond with her baby and can address some of her concerns or lack of confidence regarding child care. She may benefit greatly from joining a postpartum support group or mother-baby group.

It is crucial, at this point in therapy, that any pre-existing physical or emotional disorders be addressed. Past victimization, a poor relationship with her mother, and past abortions or miscarriages should be discussed now with the resolve to work on the issues for as long as necessary — perhaps long after the postpartum symptoms are resolved.

> *I was in therapy for about a year. There were a lot of emotional things that came out; relationships with my parents, my mother. There was a lot of stuff that had to come out. You are left with a lot of past stuff that has never really been resolved and that you've never come to an understanding of. You need to come to terms with this.*

THE THIRD PHASE OF TREATMENT

Conley calls the third stage, from four to nine months, the period of social adjustment. This period should focus on the family members individually, the couple, and the family unit. The needs of the long-suffering father should be addressed and resolved (more on this in chapter nine). Marriage counseling should be underway, if needed. Issues regarding the future of the family — such as work and child care — also can be addressed.

Termination of Treatment

The final phase, typically about nine months or later for a severe illness, is the termination of treatment. The woman can often begin withdrawal from medications. The visits to the physician and/or therapist can be terminated. The family should be educated on how to address future problems, such as the possibility of a recurrence of postpartum illness with another pregnancy.

Hospitalization

One of the most difficult decisions for the physician and family is when to hospitalize the mother. Sometimes there is no choice.

The mother who has attempted suicide or is convincingly suicidal or has tried or expressed a desire to harm her infant needs to be hospitalized, says Dr. Ricardo Fernandez, an assistant professor of clinical psychiatry at the Robert Woods Johnson/Rutgers Medical School and a postpartum expert with vast experience on treatment. "The decision regarding hospitalization of postpartum depressive patients requires a careful balance between possible disruption of the mother-child bond and imperative indications for the safety of the mother."

> *I remember being very frightened when the doctor said I might need "inpatient mental health" treatment. All I could imagine was the movie* One Flew Over the Cuckoo's Nest.

Hospitalization may also be necessary when the woman is severely dysfunctional. Family members and physicians must note, however, that it is often very difficult for a postpartum mother to accept hospitalization. She may fear that hospitalization confirms her fear that she is "going crazy." She may fear a lifetime stigma of having been admitted to a psychiatric hospital. Most important, hospitalization will severely curtail her interaction with her new baby.

Typically, the mother separated from her infant by hospitalization will have decreased opportunities for bonding with the baby. The mother may berate herself as a mother and lose all sense of self-esteem for being unable to care for her infant, says Dr. Deborah Hines, physician and postpartum expert in St. Louis, Missouri. She may feel guilty and blame herself for the illness and for abandoning her infant. Moreover, at the time of discharge, she may feel overwhelmed and unprepared to suddenly resume her role as mother.

DRUG THERAPY

In general, there are four main types of medication used to treat depression: antidepressants, monoamine oxidase inhibitors, lithium, and a new generation of antidepressants, such as the drug Prozac. In addition to these classes of drugs, minor tranquilizers are sometimes very useful in the first days of a postpartum illness when the woman has extreme anxiety and until antidepressants take effect.

Women treated for postpartum illness can expect that medications will be maintained for at least nine months. It is especially important to catch any recurrence of symptoms that might occur premenstrually or during weaning. The early termination of drug therapy is a serious problem in the treatment of depression, experts note. It is estimated that 15 to 35 percent of all patients drop out of drug treatment for depression.[4] This sometimes occurs because patients feel better. But you should keep taking your medication until the doctor says it's time to stop. You should also take care to follow your physician's directions for weaning yourself from medication.

DRUG CLASSIFICATIONS

The common antidepressants include the tricyclics and selective serotonin re-uptake inhibitors (SSRIs). Prior to the availability of the SSRIs, the most common antidepressants prescribed for postpartum depression were desipramine and nortriptyline. These classes of drugs have been in use since the late 1950s and are highly effective in many cases. The SSRIs have become popular in the 1990s. Studies tend to show that both the older and newer classes of antidepressants are equally effective, although the SSRIs typically cause fewer side effects. In general, the experts estimate that 60 to 65 percent of all depressed patients show a definite improvement with antidepressants.[5]

Antidepressants are not habit forming and are thought to work by controlling the part of the brain that controls messages between nerve cells. They can take a week or more to build up in the bloodstream and begin to work. The common side effects can include headache, insomnia, blurred vision, difficulty urinating, dry mouth, constipation or diarrhea, nausea, fatigue, weakness, and diminished sexual drive. Less common side effects are vomiting, shakiness, dizziness, and irregular heartbeat.

Tricyclic antidepressants must be used at optimal doses or they may be ineffective. The primary reason patients fail to respond to antidepressants is because they do not get adequate doses. Postpartum patients with obsessive thoughts can, in particular, require high doses of antidepressants.

Postpartum patients often also respond well to a class of drugs called monoamine oxidase (MAO) inhibitors. MAO inhibitors are often prescribed when tricyclics are ineffective. They are thought to work better in patients with anxiety or panic attacks. Experts believe they work by inhibiting nerve transmissions in the brain. These drugs need to build up in the body, and it may take a few weeks for a patient to experience the drug's full effect. Patients may need to avoid certain foods while taking MAO inhibitors, such as cheese, wine, and pickles. Side effects common with the drugs include dizziness, bladder problems, change in sexual functioning, blurred vision, drowsiness, dry mouth, constipation, and fatigue.

Postpartum patients respond especially well to serotonergic antidepressants such as fluoxetine (Prozac). A new type of antidepressant with a different chemical property, fluoxetine has distinct benefits over the older antidepressants. It is thought to work by blocking the re-uptake of serotonin in the brain. And, as has been stated, the imbalance of hormones and their subsequent influence on serotonin is considered a likely cause of postpartum illness.

The side effects associated with fluoxetine and other selective serotonin re-uptake inhibitors are fewer than those reported with tricyclics. They include nausea, tremors, drowsiness, sweating, headache, insomnia, nervousness, and diminished sexual drive. Fluoxetine can exacerbate night waking and may require sleep-inducing medication for a brief period. Unlike tricyclic antidepressants, fluoxetine can facilitate weight loss instead of promoting weight gain. This drug has been associated with reports of a sudden, acute reaction leading the patient to suicidal tendencies. But a government study failed to find any increased risk of worsened symptoms or suicide from use of this drug. Patients using medications should be carefully monitored.

Postpartum patients with anxiety and agitation may require low to normal doses of minor tranquilizers, such as the benzodiazepines: Valium, Librium, and Dalmane. The side effects include dizziness, clumsiness, and fatigue. Dr. Lee Cohen, of Massachusetts General Hospital and Harvard Medical School, notes that if there is a single symptom that distinguishes postpartum depression, it's the commingling of anxiety with the depression — a kind of agitated depression. Therefore, he often favors using antianxiety medications, such as the benzodiazepines.

Major tranquilizers, or antipsychotic drugs, are sometimes prescribed when the postpartum illness includes a manic component. A common major tranquilizer is lithium. According to Fernandez, these drugs are very beneficial to women with psychosis or mania. Because they are very strong drugs, however, the patient may be left unable to function. Fernandez has noted that mothers with postpartum depression usually require smaller doses and are much more sensitive to the side effects of major tranquilizers. Moreover, women with psychosis may respond to lower doses of antipsychotics than do nonpostpartum psychosis patients. Women with postpartum psychosis tend to have more side effects from psychotropic drugs and often require a shorter treatment course. Antipsychotic drugs can often be tapered at about two to four months of use and often can be terminated at about five or six months.

For women with obsessive-compulsive disorder, another type of medication — Anafranil — might be considered. Anafranil (clomipramine HCl) is approved for treatment of obsessions and compulsions and may be appropriate for the mother with postpartum illness who is experiencing strong OCD symptoms, such as obsessive thoughts about harming her baby. The side effects of Anafranil are similar to antidepressants and include dry mouth and drowsiness.

Sometimes it's easier to treat a postpartum patient who has a past history of a mood disorder, Cohen notes, because whatever worked for that woman in the past stands a good chance of working again. Ironically, the most guesswork is needed in treatment for the woman who only seems to have psychiatric problems in the postpartum period. "We know there is a group of women who just have episodes of postpartum depression. I'm not sure that group is adequately studied. We don't understand the best treatment for them," Cohen says.

MEDICATIONS AND BREASTFEEDING

There is much disagreement on the safety of breastfeeding and using antidepressants. Postpartum mothers who begin medication usually stop breastfeeding because of the side effects on the mother, such as drowsiness, and because of the possible effects of the drug on the infant. Other women feel very strongly that they want to continue nursing.

In some cases, breastfeeding can continue when a mother is taking an antidepressant. According to Fernandez, nursing may be acceptable if the mother is on a low-dose tricyclic. But mothers are still advised to take the medication after the baby's last feeding for the day, and then pump their breasts for the next few feedings and substitute with a bottle.

There are few studies on antidepressant treatment of nursing mothers. But the drugs nortriptyline and desipramine have been prescribed to breastfeeding mothers, and blood tests have shown no drug in the baby's blood. Experts note, however, that these tests are not as sensitive as they need to be.

In general, you should realize that all psychotropic medications are secreted in breastmilk to some degree. Except for lithium, which tends to be secreted in breastmilk in very high concentrations, "the problem is that you can't predict reliably what the concentration [of the other psychotropic medications] will be," says Cohen. "There is no data to support the safety of one antidepressant over another." In general, if a woman has done well on a particular antidepressant before pregnancy, it is usually best to remain with that medication.

Oftentimes, women on medications who opt to breastfeed will take their babies for blood tests periodically to test for concentrations of the medications in the baby's blood. "If the infant's [blood] is negative we tell mothers that it's probably OK to breastfeed but that there still may be undetectable amounts there," Cohen says.

If you want to continue to breastfeed and you, or your doctor, are concerned about the side effects of antidepressants on your nursing baby, a recent study from the University of Iowa is very reassuring. It found that women who underwent a type of psychotherapy called interpersonal psychotherapy improved significantly without the assistance of antidepressants. Interpersonal psychotherapy, which focuses on concrete problems in the patient's life, may be especially useful for women with postpartum illness, says Dr. Scott Stuart, a University of Iowa psychiatrist and researcher on postpartum disorders, because it "directly addresses issues associated with postpartum role transitions."[6]

Hormone Therapy

The medications used to treat mood disorders in postpartum women are the same as those used in people with general depression. But a treatment unique to women with reproductive-related mood disorders involves the use of hormones.

Hormone therapy, such as the use of estrogen and progesterone, has been used frequently in recent years for women with premenstrual syndrome. There is much anecdotal evidence that progesterone helps resolve many of the symptoms of PMS. But studies are not clear on whether progesterone really works in the postpartum period. Women who have worsening of symptoms premenstrually might benefit from progesterone, Fernandez says. But, he adds, "When you're dealing with progesterone, you're dealing in an area where there is very little research being done."

Cohen says that there are many anecdotal reports of women becoming worse by taking progesterone for postpartum depression. "We've seen some disastrous results. Women will describe a result that is the furthest thing from relief."

Hormone therapy deserves more research to clarify its possible benefits in postpartum illness. Treatment with an estrogen patch and antidepressants has shown promise, according to Dr. Deborah Sichel.

Electroconvulsive Therapy

Despite the range of treatment alternatives, some women with postpartum illness fail to improve adequately over the course of several months. One alternative that professionals and the patient and her family might consider at this juncture is the use of electroconvulsive therapy, or ECT.

Postpartum experts report that ECT has been highly successful in the treatment of postpartum disorders. ECT is more commonly used in Europe, but there has been much resistance to ECT in the United States.

During ECT, the patient is briefly put to sleep with an intravenous anesthetic so that the treatment is neither experienced nor remembered. A muscle relaxant is given to minimize muscle contractions. Electrodes are placed either on both sides of the scalp or on just one side of the head. A low level of electrical current is administered under careful supervision.

ECT has been used since the 1940s. In the early years, it was often used inappropriately and harshly, resulting in lingering controversy. This is unfortunate because ECT is considered a highly effective treatment for select patients; in particular, patients for whom there is little other effective treatment and whose condition might progressively become worse without some successful, rapid intervention.

ECT usually requires seven to twelve treatments. With bilateral treatment (electrodes on both sides of the scalp) patients may experience transient memory loss of events that surround the treatment. On unilateral placement, there may be less memory loss but the treatment may be less effective or require more sessions. Memory for past events or ability to learn new information is normally not affected.

ECT is coming back in favor among mental health professionals because of technological improvements such as "brain mapping" computers that monitor currents and direct the shocks to only one side of the head to reduce the chance of memory impairment. According to officials at the National Institute of Mental Health, ECT should be used only if certain conditions are met. It should be used only if the patient has been correctly diagnosed (this may require several independent medical opinions). It should be administered only under appropriate indications, such as when alternative drug treatment and other therapies have failed after an adequate trial. Finally, it should be used only after the professional, family, and patient have discussed the risks and side effects and weighed them against potential benefits.

Besides possible short-term memory impairment, side effects include fear of procedure and shame over having the procedure (due to its stigma). A family member can ask to be present during the treatment to help minimize the patient's fears. There should be no reason why a family member who has been adequately informed and educated about ECT should not be allowed to accompany the patient. The practice of having a family member present would help alleviate fears and erode the stigma surrounding ECT.

ECT can be valuable for the seriously ill patient who has agitated depression, is not responding well to drug therapy, and is in danger of harming herself. In one case, ECT was helpful to a mother who became suicidal after the birth of her fifth child. The woman had been known as a loving mother and very well-adjusted and active member of her community. She was breastfeeding her infant and refused to stop because it was so important to her. Her family agreed that if she were to stop breastfeeding she would probably try to kill herself. The mother and baby were admitted to a hospital mother-baby unit and the mother began ECT. She was able to continue breastfeeding her baby, and the treatments led to her eventual recovery.

PHOTOTHERAPY

Phototherapy, or light therapy, is a newer treatment that has been used with great success in people with a type of depression called seasonal affective disorder. These people tend to have recurrent bouts of depression during certain seasons, usually the winter months when there is less daylight.

According to Katherine Wisner, medical director of the Pregnancy and Infant/Parent Center at Western Psychiatric Institute in Pittsburgh, phototherapy might be beneficial for some postpartum patients. "In depression research now there is a great interest in the use of high-intensity light usually for low-energy, sleep-too-much, low-mood depressions that are characteristic of what we call seasonal depressions. We have a number of women in clinical work and research projects who had seasonal depressions and who had the same kind of depression after a birth.

The use of phototherapy addresses the important question of whether postpartum disorders are somehow linked to an imbalance of hormones that disrupt circadian rhythms in the postpartum period. A shift in hormones, or possibly the disruption of sleep, could cause circadian rhythm disruption. Phototherapy, it is suggested, might help restore the normal cycles of circadian rhythms.

PSYCHOTHERAPY

Psychotherapy should be part of every treatment plan for women seeking help for postpartum illness. Psychotherapy is the treatment of mental disorders through counseling. A wealth of research shows that psychotherapy, in the hands of a good therapist, is richly rewarding. Oftentimes, those who feel the worst realize the greatest gains. In addition, patients who remain in therapy for at least six months tend to benefit more than those who receive shorter courses of treatment. There are many forms or approaches to psychotherapy, which include psychoanalytical, behavioral, supportive, cognitive, feminist, interpersonal, family, and group therapy.

Although the underlying cause of postpartum illness might be biological and must be addressed, psychotherapy is also necessary to cope with the consequences of the illness. In fact, experts call the common feelings of failure, incompetence, and inadequacy the dominant themes of postpartum illness. These women are likely to view themselves as failures at mothering. They feel guilt, shame, and loss of control. Many feel undeserving of their babies or that they are being punished for previous "sins" in their lives.

Psychotherapy is also needed when the primary cause of the illness relates to social or psychological or lifestyle factors. Whether the cause is biological or social, the repercussions of postpartum illness described by Hamilton and Harberger in *Postpartum Psychiatric Illness* are typically the same for all women.

Not all types of psychotherapy are best suited for women with postpartum depression. For example, psychoanalysis, in which the woman's childhood is explored in depth, is probably not as central to her illness as more immediate events in her life.

The APA task force on women and depression recommends a combination of three therapies for depressed women. These include interpersonal therapy, feminist therapy, and cognitive/behavioral therapy.

As mentioned earlier, interpersonal therapy focuses on relationships and the development of better relationship skills to empower women. For the postpartum patient, this might include her confidence in her role as a mother. Impaired relational abilities, such as being a good mother, will have a profound negative effect on how the woman sees and values herself, APA experts say. "Women are often assigned the role of emotional caretakers who do the emotional and relational work of marriage or parenthood. Thus, women may be more likely to be responded to in a hostile or punitive manner by family and friends when they become depressed and cease to fulfill this nurturing role."[7]

Feminist therapy addresses issues such as power and powerlessness, developing egalitarian relationships, and exploring the source of depression. For the postpartum patient, this might include addressing whether her spouse is helping out enough at home since the arrival of the new baby or whether the woman fears she will be discriminated against because she has had a baby and is now a mother as well as an employee.

Cognitive-behavioral therapy offers management techniques that include understanding and identifying negative thinking and developing behavior skills to move more quickly into action and problem solving. For postpartum mothers, this therapy addresses decisions and actions the woman can make daily to restore her self-esteem and confidence in her new role as mother. According to the APA task force, women tend to think more about why they are depressed. Therapy can include activities to promote taking action, changing negative impressions, and reducing social isolation.

The value of psychotherapy with the right therapist cannot be underestimated. Psychotherapy has been found in recent studies to work just as well as popular antidepressants in patients whose illness is not severe. For patients with severe depression, medications usually work better than does psychotherapy alone. But receiving medications alone is a dangerous tactic with the postpartum patient because women in this phase of life have a tremendous need for support and education. "You don't just give the drugs and walk away," says Jeanne Driscoll. "There are lots of things going on in this family's life."

Psychotherapy is usually started immediately, even before drug therapy. Katherine Wisner says, "I never start with pharmacotherapy alone. I don't think that giving medication without the context of education and a working relationship is appropriate. I also strongly believe in a bio-psychosocial model of illness. That is, the optimal treatment is really provided with attention to biological and psychosocial interventions."

Psychotherapy should satisfy a number of important issues for you and your family, says Gruen, who has written extensively on psychotherapy during the postpartum period.

Early in therapy, the counselor can reassure the woman that postpartum illness happens to many women and is highly treatable. Counseling should address how you can get adequate rest, a good diet, and good physical care. You should begin to learn some stress reduction techniques and how to prioritize your responsibilities in order to make some time for yourself. Counseling helps the patient to form good support systems and assess the level of family support. The therapist can help you learn how to reframe negative thoughts and overcome feelings of blame and guilt. Finally, psychotherapy can be used to explore the option of medication. "Education, support, and structure are what the new parent most needs," Gruen says.

As therapy progresses, the patient should start to absolve herself of blame and become more able to understand what caused her illness. In this phase, therapy can address the symptoms and help the woman recognize her symptoms as signals of distress, Gruen says. Therapy validates the woman's feelings and helps her learn to express her feelings. She should continue to improve in understanding her thought processes and how she can avoid negative thoughts. Psychotherapy can begin to address what role her family of origin may have played in the development of the illness. The woman can also address her grief and feelings of lost time with her infant. Therapy should begin to address any unrealistic ideals of motherhood that the woman has harbored and seek to dismantle her need to be perfect and overcontrolling. Finally, work can begin on spousal or family issues, such as marriage or child behavior problems that have emerged during the course of the woman's illness.

In the final phase of psychotherapy, Gruen says, the patient and therapist should address issues of reconciliation. The woman should continue to grieve and mourn unmet expectations and recognize she cannot relive the lost time with her infant. She should begin to resolve unrealistic images she has of motherhood and develop more reasonable ones. She should be able to recognize her own feelings of discomfort and have the skills to deal with those feelings. She should address her level of self-esteem and practice self-care without guilt. Therapy should address the possibility of recurrence of depressive illness and how to cope with that possibility. The rebuilding of family relationships should continue. Women who undergo continued, regular psychotherapy should be able to resolve many important issues and learn coping strategies that will benefit them and their families for years to come.

THE QUESTION OF INSURANCE

"One of the most tragic consequences of postpartum psychiatric illness is the wrongful deprivation of insurance reimbursement for the medical and hospital expenses incurred in the treatment of the disorder," says Mark D. DeBofsky, a Chicago-based attorney who specializes in medical insurance issues. Although postpartum illness is intricately linked to an actual physical event — childbirth — many women find they will not receive insurance reimbursement for psychiatric illness unless it is clearly specified within their insurance plans. And, many Americans do not have adequate mental health insurance benefits.

The denial of reimbursement for postpartum psychiatric care is common. In a fascinating essay in *Postpartum Psychiatric Illness*, DeBofsky explains that grounds for denial are based on the fact that many major health insurance policies do not cover or drastically limit coverage of mental illness. Insurers often see mental health treatment as long term, costly, and unlikely to succeed. Thus, many avoid including it in their policies.

"The erroneous belief that mental illnesses are not 'real' and/or cannot be adequately treated contributes to the misperception by insurers, and even consumers, that mental health services are a 'bottomless pit' into which a great deal of money can be expended without any significant, concrete benefit to the patient or society," says Alan I. Leshner, an official with the National Institute of Mental Health.

DeBofsky argues that postpartum mental disorders should be covered in the same manner as any disease or illness because these disorders have a biological cause and because they relate to the physiology of pregnancy. Women can make a case for coverage based on this argument. "As a disease of the body, there can be no distinction between postpartum psychiatric illness and cardiovascular disease that causes, for example, a cerebrovascular accident or stroke."

Physicians must work with their patients to ensure insurance coverage. However, physicians may not link pregnancy to the disorder and instead follow terminology in the Diagnostic and Statistical Manual of Mental Disorders. The DSM— as you may recall — does not adequately address the relationship between pregnancy and mental illness. "This ignorance encourages insurers, who are themselves uninformed of the disorder, to refuse payment of benefits," says DeBofsky.

The refusal to pay is hugely important. In many cases, however, women are so ill that their families accept treatment and prepare to pay out of pocket, and then later — often successfully — sue insurers for payment. The more tragic repercussion from the lack of insurance coverage may be in the mild to moderate cases of depression in which a woman doesn't get help because of the cost of treatment and slips into what will be a lifetime of recurrent bouts of depression.

> *My insurance didn't pay for my psychotherapy. And it got to be such a stressor paying for it that it turned out to be much less stressful not to go. At least then we weren't worrying about being able to eat.*

Women with postpartum illness deserve — and should demand — competent treatment and coverage by health insurers. You are no less deserving of top-notch, comprehensive, and compassionate care than people suffering from cancer, heart disease, or any number of ailments.

CHAPTER EIGHT

Support for the New Mother

The severity of a new mother's illness and the timeliness of her treatment and recovery depends, to a great extent, on the people around her. These people include her husband or partner, parents, relatives, close friends, and doctor. The burden of illness on these people — especially the husband — is great indeed. But, for those families who are lucky enough to locate educational materials on postpartum illness or who encounter a local support group or who find a knowledgeable therapist, there is much to be done for the new mother that will set her on the road to recovery.

> *One of the things you lose is your sense of humor. My husband would try to joke and I was so upset. When I was better I would start to laugh at things again.*

Studies show that the mother's primary support person can quickly make things better or worse for her. For example, one study found that efforts to cheer up or reason with a depressed person by saying such things as "Look how lucky you are . . . stop feeling sorry for yourself" will backfire and cause the depression to worsen. The sadness that the depressed person feels now becomes loaded with feelings of failure and guilt over the pain she is causing those around her. This mishandling of the situation by a family member can send the depressed person into a tailspin.[1]

My husband came home to a nervous woman who fell on the floor crying. He called my mother in despair. She gave me a snap-out-of-it lecture.

"Parents, husbands, relatives say, 'Come on, what's wrong with you? Pull yourself together. You've never been like this. It's all in your mind. Don't you know better?' And there's absolutely no support from anyone who has been formerly supportive to them," says Seattle therapist Dawn Gruen. "If they're not getting what they need from those people whom they trust the most, then it's time to bring in outside professional counseling."

But understanding, tolerance, and patience from the family also become important when the new mother enters treatment, says Robert Hickman, marriage and family therapist and codirector of the Postpartum Mood Disorder Clinic in San Diego. "Any well-intentioned treatment plan is going to be undermined if you don't have the family on board."

THE IMPORTANCE OF THE SPOUSE'S SUPPORT

My psychologist suggested I needed inpatient psychiatric treatment. She wanted me to go into this hospital, and she said I could take the baby. Well, my husband had a fit. It was a few days before he had his outpatient surgery. He said, "How could you leave me when I need you? If you go that's the end of our marriage." I felt, okay, I'll just have to be strong. After that, it was like I was on my own.

Postpartum illness only magnifies a common problem in modern American society regarding the man's role in family life, says Louise B. Silverstein of New York University. In general, much heartache, stress, and arguing could be avoided if husbands could overcome the notion that they are less responsible in family life issues, she says. Fathers, by and large, do not feel compelled to participate equally in family life. "Until our culture includes nurturing and attachment as highly valued qualities in male gender-identity formation and defines child care as central to fathering, the achievement of equality within the confines of heterosexual marriage will remain elusive."

The husband's role in a postpartum illness is important for another reason, says Barbara Conley, a psychiatric social worker at Western Psychiatric Institute in Pittsburgh. It is the spouse who often gets his wife to a doctor and who must describe what she is experiencing to health professionals. The spouse's astute observations and handling of the crisis is of extreme importance.

"We start getting information from [the husband] but also at the very beginning we start giving him education so that he can support this woman," Conley says. "Many times we hear [husbands] saying 'Just pull yourself up by your bootstraps.' What [husbands] are doing when they're telling them that is they are trying to support them. So you reframe that. You tell them, if you want to be helpful, here's what you can do. . . . "

Finding Professional Help

Helping the new mother with postpartum illness starts by getting her to compassionate, understanding health professionals — when professional care is called for — and by monitoring her care to ensure that it is appropriate. Although women who become ill immediately after birth often are referred to a psychiatrist by the obstetrician, others whose illnesses are more mild or start later can, without appropriate medical intervention, remain ill for months or years.

It is not easy for the spouse and relatives to face the fact that the mother has become sad, frustrated, irritable, and anxious at a time when she is expected to be fully recovered from childbirth and enjoying her baby. "In our busy fast-paced lives, this [illness] can be inconvenient," says Patricia Neel Harberger, Mary Gleason

Berchtold, and Jane Israel Honikman, the authors of *Postpartum Psychiatric Illness.* "For too long we have been ignorant and lax regarding postpartum mental health issues. We have been impatient, judgmental, and even angry with new mothers. Often we have trivialized their cries for help."

Family members are not the only ones who have trivialized the new mother's cries for help. The entire network of health professionals who deal with a new mother and her baby as well as the mental health field should explore its responsibilities in identifying postpartum psychiatric illness and treatment of the disorder. Presently, it is a novelty for an obstetrician, family practitioner, internist, midwife, obstetrics or public health nurse, pediatrician, mental health counselor, psychologist, or psychiatrist to look for postpartum psychiatric illness within the general confines of their practices. Instead, it should be the rule.

"Women receive a great deal of attention during pregnancy, labor, and delivery, but all too soon the 'umbilical cord' is cut and they're out there on their own; perhaps needing our help more than ever before," says Dr. Deborah Sharp, a London-based physician. "We need to have a very high index of suspicion for this disorder and to ask quite probing and persistent questions in order to be certain that we can exclude it from our list of differential diagnoses."

THE RESPONSIBILITY OF THE OBSTETRICIAN

Too often the birth of the baby is seen as the end of the mother's ordeal. The six-week postpartum exam, in which many cases of depression could be spotted, is often a quick and brief assessment of the mother's reproductive health and future reproductive plans.

"Postnatal care is perfunctory with little thought or attention being paid to the mental well-being of the mother, apart from a pat on the shoulder and an assurance that all will settle down soon," says British physician Katharina Dalton in her book *Depression*

After Childbirth. "Today it is appreciated that postnatal depression ranks as the commonest and most severe complication in the six months following the birth, so it is astonishing that no one has recognized the need for lengthy postnatal care, with at least one extra postnatal examination at three to six months. This should be psychologically orientated and aimed at diagnosing the 10 percent of women with postnatal depression before the disability becomes chronic and too much damage is caused to the patient's life, her marriage, and her family."

Any prenatal care provider — whether that person is an obstetrician, family practitioner, or nurse-midwife — should frame physical health issues within the context of what motherhood means to the patient's entire life. "Beyond the traditional medical concerns of preventing sickness and death of the developing fetus and mother, the prenatal care providers should educate future parents in healthful behaviors, family planning, general knowledge of pregnancy and parenting, positive family relationships, and child development, as well as care of the newborn," suggest the authors of *A Decent Start: Promoting Healthy Child Development in the First Three Years of Life*, a report from the Carnegie Corporation of New York. "Those prenatal care providers regularly serving women at psychosocial risk should have a core set of services available within their practices." The authors advocate these services include home-health visits and parent-child educational centers. "The main thrust of both is to teach young mothers how to become effective teachers of their own children and to develop mutually beneficial mother-child relationships."

Embarrassment in discussing the emotional or psychiatric aspects of motherhood prevents many obstetricians from approaching their patients, says Sheila Kitzinger, author of *Women as Mothers*. Typically, she says, obstetricians remain stifled in their impersonal roles, and both the patient and the doctor suffer from anxiety and poor communication skills.

This is particularly tragic because most women feel a bond with their obstetricians and would confide in doctors if they felt invited to do so. One study found that information about postpartum illness provided by the patient's own doctor or nurse was more effective than classroom instruction delivered by a psychiatrist.[2]

"Obstetricians and pediatricians are the physicians who are most likely to come into contact with families after childbirth," says San Diego therapist Robert Hickman who, with his wife, Susan Hickman, a psychotherapist, helps families deal with postpartum illness. "They are in an ideal position to identify psychiatric symptoms if they are alert to the indicators. They can offer support through compassionate listening and responding with accurate information about the postpartum illnesses and by referring [women] to a psychiatrist who is informed about their causes and treatment."

The Pediatrician's Chance

I called my pediatrician to cancel an appointment for the baby. He knew me because of my older boy. He said, "Well, what's the problem?" I told him I felt like I had the flu. I told him I was having trouble sleeping. He said those are all symptoms of depression. He said, "That's not something you can snap yourself out of. You need to get help."

The pediatrician may be the professional with the greatest chance of identifying postpartum psychiatric illness. The pediatrician probably sees the mother more than any other health practitioner and can pick up on some warning signs, such as the mother's obsessing over the health of the baby; the presence of colic and the mother's reaction to it; or a woman's expressing repeated doubts about her abilities as a mother.

If the pediatrician suspects a problem, he should present his assessment to the mother and ask if she would like to seek help. While avoiding blaming the mother, the pediatrician can persuade the mother to seek help by appealing to her basic concern for her children. If the mother hesitates, the pediatrician can ask her to return to the office with her baby in a few weeks to see how she is doing. This expression of concern might open the door to further assessment or counseling or a referral. The pediatrician may eventually need to contact another family member if the mother resists seeking help and the welfare of the family becomes a serious concern.

The pediatrician has a responsibility to evaluate the depressed mother, says Dr. Edward Z. Tronick, a professor of pediatrics at Harvard Medical School who has researched infant-mother interaction. But few pediatricians ask a mother the simple question, "How are you doing?" "That's not done currently . . . [But] the pediatrician has a big advantage, because the pediatrician has an ally in the situation. And that ally is the infant."

For all new parents, but especially those with postpartum psychiatric illness, finding the right pediatrician is crucial. "A pediatrician who takes an interest in your adjustment and concerns about motherhood, who will respond to your phone calls about 'little things,' will be of much greater benefit to you and the baby than one who focuses attention solely on the baby's physical well-being," say Lyn DelliQuadri and Kati Breckenridge, authors of *The New Mother Care.* "A mother's reluctance to 'bother a busy doctor' is common, but when you need help it is absolutely necessary to know that help is available and that the doctor will be sympathetic and supportive rather than annoyed."

THE ROLE OF NURSES

Nurses may also have the opportunity to intervene and direct an ill new mother to treatment. In particular, home-health nurses, obstetrics office nurses, and pediatric nurses encounter new mothers and should know the signals of distress. In fact, says Dr. Deborah Sharp, because many obstetricians feel their responsibilities end with the birth of the baby, "it falls to those outside the mainstream of medical care to offer support to women with postnatal depression."

"The nurse is the health professional most likely to identify the postpartum depression and the one who has the most understanding about the phenomenon," says social worker Penny Handford. "More than one woman has told us they do not know what they would have done if the nurse had not listened to them and given them information about postpartum depression."

Nurses, by their very nature, can be the saviors of new mothers with postpartum illness. Nurses are valuable instigators of help because "nurses don't deal with disease per se but with the patient's and family's responses to disease and its treatment," says Dr. Ada Sue Hinshaw, director of the National Center for Nursing Research in a recent *New York Times* article.

Nurses can sometimes offer the most help to the support person caring for the patient. And, today, more nurses are turning their attention to areas of medical research untouched by (and uninteresting to) medical doctors. Nurses are the front-runners in the areas of disease prevention and health promotion, which are too often ignored by physicians.

Nurses can play an especially vital role if they are able to provide home-health visits to new mothers. Assigning a home-health nurse to visit a new mother is becoming a more common practice in the United States as more hospitals opt for early discharge programs for obstetrics patients. Home-health nurses have the opportunity to see the new mother in the mother's environment, in a confidential setting, and after she has been home for a few days. This then allows the nurse to assess the mother's emotional needs as well as physical health.

"It is this counseling role that is most important when we consider emotional reactions to childbirth. A compassionate and considerate health visit can be a great help to a depressed mother — offering her information, practical advice, boosting her self-confidence and self-esteem," says Sharp.

THE MENTAL HEALTH PROFESSIONAL

The roles of mental health professionals in managing postpartum psychiatric cases are "evolving," say Robert and Susan Hickman. By the time the new mother gets into treatment, several health professionals, including the obstetrician, psychiatrist, psychologist, and perhaps an internist or endocrinologist, may be involved in her care. The treating psychiatrist should be the overall case manager. But while psychiatrists are seen as the authorities on mental illness, "they are sometimes the least informed about the biochemical aspects of these illnesses."

Psychologists can also manage cases, although if medications are recommended, the psychologist cannot oversee this aspect of treatment. Psychologists often have the advantage of being able to see husbands and wives more frequently than psychiatrists. They can address individual, marriage, and family problems. Psychologists can play an especially valuable role in helping the husband or other family members in their efforts to support the mother and take over the child care.

Wherever the family seeks help and support, the primary goal should be to seek good information. According to Robert and Susan Hickman, "Families have a tremendous need for accurate information about the postpartum illness. The onset of symptoms is unexpected and, in most cases, is severely disruptive of normal functioning of wives and husbands. It is common for both spouses to actively seek information that can help them to make sense of the illnesses and the problems they create. . . . Accurate information can be a tremendous source of support. It gives shape and form to a mysterious and vicious intruder having a biological basis that is beyond the control of wives and husbands. It offers guidance about the direction treatment should take and the roles support people can play. It helps to allay the guilt and sense of responsibility that often surfaces as attempts to cast blame are initiated. This tendency toward self-incrimination seen in both husbands and wives has an insidious influence on marital and family adjustments during this crisis."

Spouses and family members need to seek the best professional help available — if professional help is required — and recognize what they can do for the new mother at home. Spouses, in particular, must limit themselves to what they can sensibly do, says Robert G. Logan, a Santa Barbara, California, internist whose wife suffered a postpartum depression. "Once the diagnosis is clearly established, treatment should be in the hands of a professional other than yourself," Logan advises spouses of postpartum patients. "Your input and perspective are helpful, but the responsibility for the choice of medication and overall program should not be yours."

Dealing with the Ill Mother

The people surrounding the new mother have to be noncritical, nonjudgmental, accepting, and nurturing to provide a good environment for healing. The spouse, relative, or friend caring for the mother with postpartum illness will, at times, feel helpless and frustrated. But, says Dr. Logan, "based on my own experience, I can assure you that there is much that you can do to help your spouse live through this difficult period. Most important, you need to continually reassure your spouse that she . . . will eventually recover."

It may help if the husband, relative, or friend charts the mother's good days and bad days and records her feelings. This can help the doctor or therapist determine her progress and allow the new mother to see that she is making progress, Dalton says.

> *The days I knew my babysitter was coming, I wasn't anxious. She was just there for a few hours. But I knew I could rest and I wasn't by myself. If someone was there it was okay. When I was alone I was terrified.*

"Relatives and friends need to have an infinite supply of patience and understanding. This applies especially to husbands, who may find it all beyond their comprehension and feel they cannot condone illogical behavior," says Dalton.

Within the basic framework of love, acceptance, reassurance, and patience, there are some dos and don'ts that will help guide the spouse or relative:

- Don't try to reason with the patient by saying such things as, "Look at how beautiful the baby is. How can you be sad?" or "Of course you won't hurt the baby. Don't worry about it."
- Don't bring attention to the new mother's shortcomings, failures, disheveled appearance, or unfinished jobs.
- Do try to understand the new mother's special needs, such as the need to rest.
- Do encourage the new mother to partake in activities during the day, such as going to a movie or out for a walk, even if she rejects suggestions. You can even gently pressure her to do so. But recognize that a depressed person is often unable to tolerate much activity.

Besides trying to avoid doing the wrong things, there are many positive actions you can undertake to promote the new mother's wellness, say experts from the Pacific Post Partum Support Society:[3]

- Give the new mother room to make whatever decisions she can make. Recognize that it is difficult for her to make decisions right now, and support and praise her choices.
- Encourage her to take one day at a time. Discourage her from dwelling on what has happened in the past or what might happen in the future. Think about the present.
- Help her to redefine who she is. Allow the new mother to talk about how the baby has changed her and how she is different from the person she used to be. Identifying what has been lost will allow her to regain her identity.
- Encourage her to give herself credit. She will feel like a failure and guilty about her shortcomings. Point out realistic goals

and acknowledge all that she has done. Remind her that being a mother is hard work.

- Share your experiences. If you are a mother, sharing what you feel will be helpful.
- Reassure her that a lack of sexual interest is normal at this time.
- Emphasize the temporary nature of her illness.
- See that she has regular, good meals.

ANTICIPATING WHAT THE NEW MOTHER NEEDS

Many mothers have a hard time accepting help, especially from their husbands, says Dr. Martin Greenberg, author of the book *The Birth of a Father.* In addition, the new mother must accept that her husband will parent differently than she does and has the right to do so. Moreover, the new mother must accept her husband's offer of help, or ask him to help if he has not stepped in to do so.

Even among healthy mothers, the first few months after childbirth are exhausting. The new mother is hard on herself, demands perfection, overreacts, and feels like she must do everything. As a result she can become fatigued, overwhelmed, irritable, tense, and quick tempered.

"Why is it so hard for new parents to admit, 'I need help?' Perhaps it is because accepting help seems like admitting failure ... It is ironic that it is often the parent who needs relief most urgently who most vehemently protests against it," Greenberg says. "There may be times, however, when despite her clear need for relief, your wife is reluctant to let you take over. . . . [The spouse's] role at such a time can be crucial. It is in these pressured circumstances that you can provide the help that may save the day."

Greenberg calls relieving the mother from child care "spelling" and offers some guidelines for spelling:

1. Discuss the concept beforehand and the fact that each of you will require relief now and then.

2. Spelling should be nonjudgmental.
3. Spelling shouldn't focus on the difficulties the caretaking parent is experiencing.
4. Work out a signaling system in advance, like a nod or gesture from the parent who is asking to take over. This relieves the situation from becoming one in which the husband says, "Why don't I take the baby?' and thus sounds critical of the mother.

"To your wife, your verbal comments, even when made in the most neutral fashion, can sound like a criticism of her mothering ability and result in an angry response," Greenberg says. "She is already angry and critical of herself. Those continued shrieks of the baby, despite her best efforts, result in an increase in her self-doubts, and with this comes a vulnerability to feeling criticized."

TALKING AND LISTENING

The most important role support people play is that of encouraging the new mother to express her feelings and of listening to her in a supportive and nonjudgmental manner. Accept the new mother's feelings. Remind her that if she can express and accept feelings, that is a step toward healing.

Women who are feeling very irritable and frustrated may believe that they are going to be bitter and angry for the rest of their lives. Women will commonly respond to this fear by trying to bury unpleasant feelings. "But censoring them has the opposite effect to what was intended because it usually prolongs the feelings. What helps is to air your angry feelings," say experts from the Pacific Post Partum Support Society.[4]

Women with postpartum illness also avoid expressing their feelings for fear that others will disapprove of them. "Fear of disapproval by friends and family members, particularly husbands, prevents self-disclosure. An atmosphere of unconditional acceptance of the new mother's postpartum emotional experiences is imperative. Fear of rejection is a most formidable barrier to seeking help," say Harberger, Berchtold, and Honikman in *Postpartum Psychiatric Illness.*

It is the difficult task of the support person to recognize when the new mother is holding something back and then to encourage her to reveal what is on her mind, says Nancy Berchtold, founder of the support group Depression After Delivery. This can be critical when early symptoms of the disorder have just begun to emerge. "Those who surround the new mother must be sensitive to the many ways she cries out for help. Too often these cries are not heard."

When the new mother does express her feelings, listen in a noncritical way, accepting whatever the new mother chooses to tell you. Remember that she may act paranoid and may not trust your intentions of helping her.

> *I went to my parent's house for lack of places to go. I didn't know what to do. I called friends for advice. With my anxiety at an all-time high and my distrust at an all-time high, it was difficult to listen to anyone.*

The ill mother often feels that she will never get well and that her future is doomed. "Whenever they express these feelings [of hopelessness and failure], the healthy spouse should listen supportively — even if it taxes his . . . patience — to indicate understanding of how the depressed spouse feels," says Dr. Robert Logan. "It is useless and inadvisable to contradict negative statements, for they are often based to some extent on facts: The depressed spouse really cannot function effectively in the usual roles. The response should therefore be positive, reassuring, and supportive."

Don't worry about what you are going to say to the new mother. You don't need to have all the answers. "Listening to her without criticizing is much more important than saying the 'right' thing or having all the answers," say experts from the Pacific Post Partum Support Society.[5]

Try to avoid expressing your own fears or reacting with distress to what the new mother is saying. Present a calm demeanor as you listen and empathize. "Do allow the new mother to talk freely and express her innermost fears without showing shock or amazement," Dr. Katharina Dalton says. "Often there are no grounds for her fears, but let her speak about them, she needs to get them out of her system. Do show consideration and sympathy for her in her predicament."

Allowing the Mother to Care for her Child

It is important that the family or friends of the new mother provide a safe environment for both the mother and child or children. The family should not allow the mother to be alone with the baby if there is any chance she might harm it or herself, Dalton says.

But, in the case of the mother who is acutely ill, it can be very difficult to determine just how much of the child care she should be encouraged or allowed to undertake. Except in cases in which the threat of harm to the baby is quite serious — and the health professional should help the family determine this — the new mother should be allowed to care for her child as much as she wants to and is able to. Recognize that often the new mother cannot care for the new child and doesn't want to. In these cases, it is helpful for friends or relatives to take over child care. But each day, be open to the possibility that the mother may be ready to start assuming some child care responsibilities again as she begins to recover.

Because the new mother's self-esteem is usually quite low at this point, being able to care for the baby can help her adopt a better attitude about herself. For this reason, hospitalization should be avoided if at all possible.

"We like to keep the woman with the child even if she can't take care of the child," says Barbara Conley. "Most of our women want very much to take care of their child and want to be the only one doing it. So we tell Grandma, 'It's okay if you don't do any-thing but sit there in the house and watch her try to take care of the children if that is what she wants to do.'"

Sometimes, Conley says, the mother may just be frightened to be in the house by herself. In this case, the support person can merely sit and keep her company. Too often, well-meaning people take over the child care and the mother is too demoralized to assert her desire to take care of the children, say Mary Ann Krause and E. Scott Redman of Wright State University. "In these cases it will be useful to have relatives back off and restore the new mother's control over infant care." Sometimes, hiring a babysitter or nanny works well because it allows the new mother to direct child care activities and restores her control over the situation.

THE SUICIDAL CRY

Very few mothers with postpartum disorders think about, discuss, or attempt suicide. But family members and support persons need to be aware of the signs and symptoms of suicidal behavior and know how to react if the situation arises.

Support groups for postpartum illness have issued detailed guidelines to their telephone volunteers on how to deal with suici-dal calls. Friends and relatives may also find these guidelines useful:

- Try to be positive by emphasizing the person's most desirable alternatives.
- Try to sound calm and understanding.
- Emphasize the temporary nature of the person's problems.
- Encourage the person to talk about her feelings.
- Reinforce the person by praising what she does well.
- Don't sound shocked.
- Don't talk about what shock and embarrassment a suicide would cause the family.
- Don't debate the person.

- Don't reject the person's feelings.
- Always call a doctor if you have any doubts about the mother's safety or your ability to protect her.

Suggestions for the New Mother

If your experience with postpartum depression is severe, you need to rely heavily on those around you for help. If your illness is milder, you also need support and reassurance. But, if you have the ability to act on your own behalf, don't wait around for the support or permission of others to seek help.

A good place to start is by lowering your expectations of yourself. For some reason, women who have babies seem to feel that they should do more, be more, and want more when they have a baby, instead of realizing that this great new responsibility requires cutting back on what they can achieve. If you can direct your attention on the wonder of your beautiful child and worry less about everything else around you, you will feel less stressed and much happier. And so will everyone else around you.

"High expectations of oneself usually lead to high expectations of others," say experts with the Pacific Post Partum Support Society. "You may expect your 2-year-old to behave in ways which are unrealistic for such a young child. When the child cannot meet your standards you may feel like a failure as a mother. As you start to lower these expectations of yourself, you will become more accepting both of your own limitations and those of others."

When you bring home a new baby, the feeling of losing control, losing a part of yourself and your freedom, may be so overwhelming that you may cling to that which you know you can still control: your house, your work, and your relationships.

But look around and ask yourself: What can I let go today without consequence? Is it really necessary to expect the toddler to be toilet trained? Is it really important that the house is dusted?

Must I enroll the five-year-old in dance lessons this month or can it wait until summer?

Force yourself into lowered expectations by picking out one or two very manageable tasks per day to accomplish. Build up as you are able to do so. Lowering your expectations includes recognizing that you will not be a perfect parent and that it is fine to be an imperfect parent. As mentioned earlier, recognize that you can be a "good enough" mother. Your baby will forgive you for mistakes.

"There is no formula for good mothering except that it achieves a balance between the needs of the mother and the child. No one will argue that it is difficult to be sensitive to a child when you are fatigued, ill, depressed, preoccupied, or otherwise under stress. Only when you are healthy and free from stress can you do your job well and like it. So amid your concern and effort to fulfill your child's needs, remember that you need much, too," say DelliQuadri and Breckenridge in *The New Mother Care*.

Indeed, one of the hardest things about being a mother is learning that to take good care of your children you must take very good care of yourself. "Perhaps the most important task that we set for a mother is that she start doing things for herself rather than just for her family," says Penny Handford. "We ask the mother to find time in her day for at least one break from her mothering duties."

Take a bath, have coffee with a friend, take a nap, or wander around a mall and buy something for yourself. This use of time can be especially difficult for you if you are on a maternity leave and are scheduled to return to work in a few weeks. You may feel you should be spending every moment with your infant.

But, Handford says, "Getting a babysitter is often a turning point for a mother because the woman is saying that she deserves to have time for herself — to pay the money for a babysitter — and is finally able to be assertive enough to carry it through."

If you do not have someone in your home who can invite you to express your feelings and can listen to you objectively and patiently — and many women do not — look outside your immediate circle for someone who can — perhaps a friend, an older woman who has many years of mothering experience, or a therapist. Buy a notebook and write down your feelings.

> *When I had postpartum depression I would write things down that bothered me and would tell myself, "I'll deal with them in the morning." I couldn't let go of things. But the fact that I wrote them down helped me to let go of them. In the morning, I would look at that and think, "that's no big deal."*

Don't deny your feelings or your right to express them. There is nothing shameful, wrong, or bad about experiencing a postpartum illness. Unfortunately, some women have a habit of silencing their feelings. This can be harmful in a postpartum illness. New mothers need to know that expressing their doubts or negative feelings about parenthood is as important as expressing the joys.

Remember that crying is cathartic. "Since tears can be healing and actually relieve stress, we encourage the women to view their grief and sadness as acceptable feelings and to allow their expression," Handford says.

Recognize what a great physical task pregnancy and childbirth is and give yourself time to recover physically. The obsession with getting back to prepregnancy weight is very unfortunate for all women, especially for depressed women.

Moreover, say experts with the Pacific Post Partum Support Society, "When a woman is depressed she often either overeats or feels that she cannot eat at all."[6] Don't blame or chastise yourself for overeating. Don't worry about your dress size now. You will eat better and look better as you begin to feel better.

DEALING WITH FRIGHTENING SITUATIONS

Some women with postpartum illness have thoughts of harming themselves or their babies or imagine morbid things happening to their loved ones. The majority of women with obsessive thoughts will not harm their babies. And, as discussed previously, these thoughts are part of the illness and cannot be controlled.

If you are having bizarre, disturbing, uncontrollable thoughts, don't berate yourself. You are not bad, evil, or possessed. Remember that these thoughts don't represent reality. Tell yourself that having a scary thought is not the same as acting on it. You will not harm the baby. If you can, get away from your children when you have a scary thought. Put the baby in a safe place, such as the crib or infant swing, and go to another room. Cry, take a bath, eat. Don't try to control your thoughts or fight the image. Find someone to talk to. Some women are helped by imagining their thoughts are on a tape and they are cutting the tape or they are using an eraser to wipe out the image. Pretend your thoughts are on TV and change the channel.

"Try always to remember that the fantasies are only thoughts and feelings which arise because you are in a very stressful situation right now," say Pacific Post Partum Support Society experts. "They are a common part of a postpartum depression and do not mean that you are going crazy."[7] Also, remember that obsessive thoughts can be worse at night or when you are tired.

CONSERVING ENERGY

Rest is a key ingredient to recovering your health. Look for energy drains, for example, too much coffee, bothersome friends or relatives, isolation, inactivity, too little help, and too many responsibilities. Recognize these energy drains and take action to change them. Watch yourself for signs of tension, for example, clenched jaw, tense shoulders, stiff neck, knotted stomach, and the presence of nervous habits. Spot the signs and tell yourself to relax.

Don't rush. Make a concerted effort to slow down. Don't run when you hear the baby crying. Focus on what you are doing.

Don't think about the next task. Complete one thing at a time. This is not the time to make lists and check them off. The best advice may be to relish good times with your infant. When your baby is content and snuggled up next to you and you have made eye contact, let everything else go. You will never look back and regret the precious moments you spent with your baby. Neither will you regret not having kept up the house perfectly.

Accept all the help you can get. If friends offer, say yes and tell them how they can help. Ask if they can babysit or run an errand or take older children off your hands for a few hours.

Ask your own mother for help if you are inclined to do so. "For many women, the struggle for independence and an identity distinct from their mothers' makes if difficult to ask for emotional support and help during childbearing," says DelliQuadri and Breckenridge. "But you should be assured that you are not regressing if you need your mother at the time you bear your own child."

The new mother should remind herself not to take on any added responsibilities in the postpartum period, such as moving, helping out relatives or friends in need, or remodeling the house. Try to take as much time as you need and can afford away from your job outside the home. Conversely, return to work if you feel pressured at home. Do things to please yourself. Remember to do things with your spouse, as a couple, apart from the children. Exercise if you enjoy it. Finally, look for support groups and resources in your community that can assist you.

Support Groups

In September 1985, after suffering her own postpartum depression, Nancy Berchtold of Morrisville, Pennsylvania, began the first postpartum support group in the United States, calling it Depression After Delivery (DAD). Five women attended the first meeting. Berchtold decided the message of the group would simply be: You're not alone.

Berchtold's founding of DAD has been the most significant development toward understanding postpartum psychiatric illness in more than a century. In the void left by the medical field's ignorance of this important issue, DAD has stepped in and ignited a grass roots movement among mothers. This movement is primarily aimed at women helping each other. But it also focuses on promoting awareness of postpartum illness and encouraging more medical research and social understanding.

In its short existence, DAD has fielded many thousands of information requests or calls for help. The organization has expanded to 80 support groups and has 250 telephone volunteers. DAD has also sent out hundreds of information packets to professionals. When DAD members appeared on the *Phil Donahue Show* in 1988, they heard from 520 people. A mention in a 1990 Ann Landers column elicited a response from 2,619 people.

"We are the light in the darkness for so many families," Berchtold says. "In some cases, the support groups are their first link in getting help."

Consider the sampling of letters she has received from families in need:

We went to twenty different agencies for help and none understood at all.

• • •

My wife keeps saying that she wants to die. And I keep saying that you don't want to die, you just want to get better. Can you do anything to help us?

Not all support groups for women with postpartum illness fall under the organizational framework of DAD. Nevertheless, most support groups operate in a similar fashion and provide a very important service. The mother finds she is not the only one to have this disorder. These groups offer support, hope, information, education, development of interpersonal skills, and catharsis for repressed feelings.

"Groups are necessary from a number of vantage points: the person suffering the illness no longer feels isolated; the partner receives encouragement, support, and information about the illness and what he can do to assist the new mother; the mother can ask questions that she may be afraid to ask her physician," say Nancy Berchtold and Melanie Burrough (also of Depression After Delivery). It is important to remember, though, that "support groups are never a substitute for a doctor's care."

Support groups can act like group therapy. "The most successful new mothers in therapy groups learn to be more trusting, open, and honest; to give and accept forthright feedback," Berchtold and Burrough say.

Most important, women learn how common postpartum disorders are. "People share a common sorrow and tragedy. And along with that comes hope, because many people in the support group have survived the illnesses and are doing well. You have examples of women who are proof that you can get through this," Berchtold says.

Support groups can be located by calling DAD or Postpartum Support International, a worldwide postpartum informational organization. Hospitals are a good place to look for a postpartum support group or to start one. The fact that early discharge is encouraged by insurers should provide incentive for hospital administrators to consider sponsoring a group.

Support groups are not for everyone. Initially, a very ill mother may not be able to attend a support group. Likewise, mothers with very mild postpartum depression or blues may feel that the group she is attending has more serious concerns. Some women are simply not helped by talking to other depressed women. The American Psychological Association National Task Force on Women and Depression found that women may intensify depression by gathering to talk over their feelings. According to Dr. Ellen McGrath, chairwoman of the group, "If a woman is very depressed, it's not that helpful to talk over those feelings with another woman, because they can become partners in depression for each other. It's as though the depression were contagious." McGrath concluded that a more effective approach was for a depressed woman to take some positive step toward changing circumstances that are part of the depression or getting therapy.[8]

"Self-help groups may not fit a person's personality," Berchtold says. "Over the years, I've seen women come to the support group once. We ask them to try it twice. We say don't give up the first time because every meeting is different. But some women say that to hear the stories of other women made them more agitated, more anxious. It was comforting to know other women had the same feelings, but that, at that point, they just couldn't cope. But I think [support groups] are for the majority." Hearing other women's experiences often relieves a woman of her own guilt and fear.

> *When I went to the support group I talked to other women who were taking antidepressants. I have such a hang-up about drugs. I just had this aversion to it. I thought that's a real admission of failure. But here I was talking to these women whom I could identify with — professional women — and they were taking medications. So it must be okay.*

Says Susan Hickman: "There is nothing more therapeutic than hearing other women talk about their own experience and their own symptoms. That normalizes the experience for the mother."

CHAPTER NINE

The Effects of Postpartum Illness on the Family

When a postpartum mother becomes ill, you can be sure that her husband, infant, other children, and perhaps close relatives and friends will be affected — sometimes dramatically so. The insidious aspect of postpartum psychiatric illness is that it will — eventually if not immediately — encompass the entire family, sometimes creating a morass of problems much bigger than the illness itself. Postpartum disorders inevitably cause "unhappiness and disruption of marriages, families, and homes," says British physician Katharina Dalton.

There are three primary considerations regarding postpartum illness and its effects on the family:

1. How the illness affects the marriage
2. How the illness affects the mother's primary support person (usually the husband)
3. How the illness affects the infant and older children

THE MARRIAGE: IN SICKNESS AND IN HEALTH

The birth of a baby is disruptive to any marriage, even when both partners are healthy, and even when the pregnancy was wanted. The postpartum period is, normally, a time of readjustment in a marriage, a time of renegotiating roles. A strong marriage survives the baby and comes out stronger. A marriage with problems, research shows, almost inevitably suffers.

Marriage counselors have identified several common sources of conflict between spouses when a new baby enters the family:

- One parent feels overlooked or ignored. "The infatuation with the baby often leaves one of the spouses out," says Seattle family therapist Dawn Gruen. "Twosomes become threesomes, but someone gets left out."
- The couple experiences financial pressures, especially if the new mother has left her job.
- The couple fails to renegotiate household and parenting responsibilities. The unequal sharing of household and family tasks is the most likely cause of marital conflict.

New parents often overlook the need to talk out their feelings. New mothers don't like to admit that motherhood is not as glamorous or enchanting as it was cracked up to be; nor do new parents like to admit that to each other. There is a sort of conspiracy of silence between partners about the hardships of parenting.

"They don't end up being very honest about what is difficult for them," Gruen says. "There is a lot of isolation, and there is a lot of fear that 'This is the way it's going to be for the rest of my life.'"

In addition, both parents feel tired, overwhelmed, and wholly undertrained. "Men are just as anxious and confused about handling the baby," Gruen says. "Nobody expects the highs and the lows. The intensity of the rage." If you add postpartum illness to these normal adjustment issues, a family can be devastated.

MARRIAGE AND POSTPARTUM ILLNESS

Studies show that marital stress is a major problem of postpartum illness, says San Diego therapist Robert Hickman in *Postpartum*

Psychiatric Illness. A 1988 study found that anxiety and depression in the husband were the principal reactions to a wife's postpartum illness. "[The illness] affects families, their lifestyles, and their hopes and dreams," Hickman says. "The changes are dramatic and sometimes devastating." When a couple are married, the love and the commitment they feel . . . instills a confidence that they'll be able to deal with whatever comes up." But postpartum illness, which many new parents may have never even heard of — let alone expected — is among the greatest of challenges.

> *If somebody would have told me when my wife first got sick what was to come, I don't know if I could have handled it. But we learned to take it one day at a time.*

And although a couple may fear a birth defect or Sudden Infant Death Syndrome when they are expecting a child, "no one expects something will happen to the woman. It's this out-of-the-blue quality that makes this experience devastating," Hickman says. "The causes are unknown [to the couple]. It's totally baffling, and the usual coping mechanisms families use are ineffective. And this leads to severe stress that can become overwhelming and overpowering."

Couples who do not seek help for their marriage or family unit face a high risk of divorce from postpartum illness, Gruen says. "Marriages — many of them — going through postpartum depression, end up dissolving. Or the trauma is so severe it ends up lasting the rest of their lives. Putting back together the family after the crisis is important, renewing those bonds. Learning to trust each other again and work together."

Some couples stay together and adapt for better or for worse. Hickman adds: "What we find is that the changes strike at the weakest points of the relationship."

> *A couple of weeks after the baby was born, we had a fight about the dog. The dog is 45 pounds, and I*

wanted the dog out of the room with the baby. Well,
that was one more change too many for him. I took
the baby and went to my mom's house. I was angry
with my husband. I knew I needed sleep. I hadn't
slept in two and a half weeks. I called a friend from
the church who is a lawyer and said I wanted a
divorce. He knew something was wrong with me.
He said, "You need to go to the hospital."

The inability to deal with the illness, especially in the early stages, can send a marriage to rock bottom long before the woman even gets medical help. The father, particularly, often denies that his wife is ill, or seriously ill. Knowing he feels this way, the wife may also try to deny her illness or fear telling her husband how she truly feels.

Other times, the father tries to be strong and attempts to cheer up his wife. He is the optimist and she is the pessimist, say Mary Ann Kraus and E. Scott Redman of Wright State University in a report on postpartum illness. "The more encouraging he becomes, the more discouraged and hopeless she becomes. He cannot speak out about his fears and she cannot contradict him."

When at last the illness becomes undeniable, the husband usually takes one of two courses of action: He withdraws from the family or he takes over his wife's role. If he withdraws, by staying at work longer or by finding excuses not to go home, this devastates the woman. The new mother is alone, isolated, unsupported, and, perhaps, in danger of harming herself and her child.

On the other hand, if the husband assumes his wife's responsibilities for household tasks and child care along with his own duties, both partners can quickly become resentful of the situation. "The more of her work he does, the more lost and like a failure she feels and she starts to resent him," say the authors of "Post Partum Depression and Anxiety," a booklet written by the members of the Pacific Post Partum Support Society. "At the same time the husband or partner starts to resent his wife for not coping as well as he thinks she should. A 'no-win' cycle develops and puts a great strain on the relationship."

I think I was more mad at her than anything. She wasn't paying attention about what she was supposed to be doing. She wasn't getting her act together. I had never heard about things like this [postpartum illness] at all.

Anger is a common emotion in a home where postpartum illness has crept in. In some cases, the husband may verbally abuse his wife. And because the woman with postpartum illness is already down on herself, she may accept this assault, feeling she has caused and deserves it.

HELP FOR THE MARRIAGE

There are, of course, many very successful strategies for coping with, and conquering, the part of postpartum illness that targets the marriage. Couples do survive and end up stronger and more united after the illness.

I don't know what made him so sensitive and smart and know the right thing to say. I just thank God. Without him, I don't think I would have made it. Now, I think both of us feel that life is short.

The key element is educating the family about the illness, says Hickman. Education instills hope and reduces stigma. If the family goes together for the initial medical assessment and/or undertakes family or marriage therapy in addition to the mother's individual treatment, "it promotes a shared understanding of what the illness is and what is the best way to treat it."

It can also be useful for the husband to participate in his wife's therapy — even if it's just listening — because he can later remind and clarify for her what was discussed. This is important when she is experiencing confusion during the acute phase of depression. When the illness is severe or protracted, it's especially important that the couple acquire a new set of skills and a new way of doing things, at least until the mother has recovered.

I always tried to joke around and tease her when she was in a bad mood. But that didn't work with this.

Experts stress that the couples' ability to tell each other how they feel is crucial. "Communicating, even about conflict, is an opportunity for bringing you closer," say DelliQuadri and Breckenridge, authors of *The New Mother Care.* "Backing away leaves the distance between you to be filled with anger and resentment."

Couples enduring a postpartum illness should take one day at a time and not worry about the future or the past. Sometimes it even helps to adopt an experimental attitude toward problem solving, experts say.

Our baby has colic. And in the beginning, my husband was helpful. Now it's to the point where he's saying "Let's move on . . . Let's get a babysitter . . . Let her cry." I don't know what to do. I feel like every time she cries I have to pick her up.

Families should not attempt to make any big decisions at this time. When the new mother is extremely ill, it is common for either partner to react hastily, sometimes separating, seeking a divorce, or committing the mother to an institution. When a new mother first appears for treatment of a postpartum illness, Barbara Conley asks the family to enter the period she calls "suspended animation." Conley, a psychiatric social worker at the Pregnancy and Infant/Parent Center at Western Psychiatric Institute in Pittsburgh, says, "This is to allow time to wait until treatment can start taking effect. Many times, the distraught husband brings his ill wife in to a therapist's office and proclaims: 'I just want a divorce.' We say, 'Just wait. This is what is going on. This may be what you want to do. But don't do it now.' And I usually make them a bargain . . . Sometimes I'll say, 'Give me four weeks. And then we'll talk about this.'"

Later in recovery, the couple can backtrack and discuss what has happened. According to Gruen, some actions the couple in recovery might take include:

- Accept the illness as a learning experience, an opportunity for growth.
- Avoid trying to control the other's rescue attempts. Stop taking over for each other.
- Diminish the sick role and give the father a voice. "Men are afraid of trusting that they can say how angry they are and how fearful they are."
- Restrain from a too-rapid recovery.
- Stress the importance of communication.
- Remind each other that bad days today are not as bad as they were three months ago.
- Address their feelings of grief and loss over what has happened in their lives.
- Address how each needs to take care of herself or himself.

THE PLIGHT OF THE FATHER

Beyond the intricate effects on the marriage, postpartum illness puts a severe individual and highly personal strain on the father. He can be overwhelmed with unexpected feelings. One study found that 13 percent of men sampled felt depressed at some time during the eight weeks after the birth of their first baby.[1] Another study found that 62 percent of men experience some postpartum depression at some point in the four months after the birth of the baby.[2]

Part of the father's distress may have to do with his tendency to identify with his wife, studies show. "His psychic reality is that he, too, is pregnant and is creating something inside himself . . . Since a father's fantasy of the pregnancy is similar in many respects to the mother's he may have similar reactions to the delivery," say doctors Stuart Asch and Lowell Rubin, psychiatrists who performed this research while at the Mount Sinai School of Medicine in New York.

Research shows that fathers, too, can suffer from postpartum depression related to their fears of fatherhood, anxieties, loss of freedom, financial pressures, insecurities, and stress. Like new mothers, new fathers commonly experience a feeling of confusion, says Dr. Martin Greenberg, author of *The Birth of a Father*. Some men feel fatherhood thrusts them into a dream world. They feel dazed.

"But it's not a dream," Greenberg says. "And as your sense of unreality persists, you may begin to feel a kind of isolation and confusion about your role now that your baby is home. What do you do as a father? Of course, your work is an important contribution, but you did that before. So what will you do differently now? Don't be alarmed at your feelings. This is simply a confusing time, when your sense and even your view of the world are in disarray."

Some men feel conflicted about becoming fathers and fear they won't be a good role model for the child, Gruen says. Some men find they view the baby less positively than they expected.

> *I think he was going through something himself after the baby was born. The adjustment to the insanity at home . . . Going into this pregnancy, he had an industrial accident and lost his job. I was supporting the family. I realized that we had been going through a lot. But we've made it this far. When I realized that, it melted away a lot of my resentment. I felt, we have to be united and keep each other strong. I also recognize he's limited in what he can give me.*

Like new mothers, new fathers may be shocked by the demands of parenting and how life has changed. And, like new mothers, fathers are not expected to discuss the difficulties or negative aspects of becoming a parent.

The man whose wife suffers from a postpartum psychiatric illness faces a huge burden of other problems and concerns in addition to these "normal" issues. "New fathers often react with confusion, shock, denial, and anger. They too have subscribed to the myth of blissful parenthood and are likely to be ill-prepared for the demands placed upon them," say Harberger, Berchtold, and Honikman in *Postpartum Psychiatric Illness.*

Fathers feel they have lost control of their home life and are powerless, says Gruen. "This is not what they expected would happen. The fear of having his spouse not functioning at all can be overwhelming for them."

The father is often dismayed, even terrified, to see his beloved wife incapacitated. Greenberg notes that some men hang on to an image from their childhood of the loving, all-giving mother. It can be hard for them to accept their own wife as an imperfect or incapacitated mother. "Our image of our mothers is distorted by time and our needs," he says. "But if you remember your own mother as loving, always there when you wanted or needed her, you may want to perpetuate that all-caring image. If you remember her as never or rarely there when you needed her, you may have been searching for some time to find a replacement. With your wife's emergence now as a mother, there is an increasing tendency to elevate her to the position of the great mother."

Many men fear the illness will last indefinitely and that life will never be normal again. They may find that their former coping skills don't work in the face of this overwhelming illness.

> *The hardest time for me was watching her go through it. The depression has been a lot worse. When the psychosis is over, it's over.*

"It's very devastating when what they used to know worked doesn't work any more," Gruen says. "In many couples the woman was the caretaker; she took care of the man, both emotionally and physically. All of a sudden he's doing everything. It's really a switch from being cared for in many ways to being the primary caretaker; coming home from work and being there for everyone."

*I was worried my husband wouldn't stay with
me. Here I gave him a baby and he lost me. He felt
helpless and frustrated because he didn't know
what to do.*

Many men simply do not know how to be supportive, say San
Diego therapists Robert and Susan Hickman. They have not
learned to be supportive; nor have they been socialized to do so.
They consider this role effeminate. "When forced to assume a role
that is both extrinsic and threatening to their self-image, many
husbands begrudgingly or hesitatingly perform the necessary tasks.
These conditions also contribute to a husband's feeling victimized
and frustrated."

Many men may also feel uncomfortable facing or discussing
painful, personal experiences that relate to family relationships,
such as a postpartum depression. They discover that it's very difficult to hear what the wife is saying and then respond lovingly.
"Outpourings of emotion are traditionally very threatening for
men to hear at a time when compassionate listening and responding are needed," the Hickmans say.

The father commonly is angry over this unexpected turn of
events. He is angry over the change in his spouse. He is angry that
this postpartum time — which was supposed to have been so special — has become a nightmare. He is angry at health professionals, perhaps his wife's doctor, for not informing or warning the
couple that postpartum illness was a possibility. He is angry at the
baby for disrupting his life.

Moreover, the father, too, eventually becomes exhausted. A
surge of initial support often dissolves into anger and resentment
as he becomes exhausted caring for his wife and baby. He finds
his resolve to see the family through this crisis fading. "If she has
one good day they want to wipe [the experience] out. They want
to say she's okay now, let's get on with our lives," Gruen says.

The father may deny that the wife is ill or refuse to face her symptoms. And, usually, most men have no clue about how to address the

situation. They have no idea what kind of doctor or health facility to take the mother to. "When you look at the father's experience, he's even more in the dark and ignored," says Nancy Berchtold of DAD.

"Most of the people I see have never been to a counselor," Gruen says. "It's very foreign to them not to use their own resources to deal with things."

Hickman, who counsels men whose wives suffer from postpartum psychiatric illness, says there are five predominant problems for men:

1. Family relationships are strained. The father must become the primary caregiver. He becomes tense because of his increased responsibilities. He may interpret his wife's unresponsiveness as a sign of personal rejection.

2. Medical concerns arise. Husbands are often left with the task of trying to find good medical care and of being the key person to describe symptoms during the initial medical assessment. Some unlucky families stumble into the hands of health care providers who are uninformed or not up to date on postpartum illness. So, if the illness persists, the husband may be unable to understand why. He may accuse the wife of malingering or may start to deny the seriousness of the illness. "This could lead a wife to hide her distress from her husband," Hickman notes, "which will only make the situation worse."

3. Financial concerns arise. This is a huge problem, especially if long-term psychiatric care or hospitalization is needed.

4. Family activities and plans are curtailed. The husband's leisurely weekly golf or tennis outing may be set aside, which can leave him no outlet for stress reduction, relaxation, and escape.

5. Social relationships suffer. The family may find that friends are put off by the illness and the mother's "strange" behavior. Relatives might fail to understand and be critical of the illness. Sometimes, even relatives who are trying to be supportive can become a nuisance.

Help for the Father

The burden for fathers increases with the length of the illness. "Ultimately, the family becomes exhausted," Gruen says. "Members who have been initially supportive can become resentful as emotional resources are depleted. The father can be debilitated by the tension of being called home from work at any time, of arranging for 24-hour care in some cases, and of dealing with a confusing situation."

Ironically, when the mother finally does begin to recover, the father often falls apart. The father has really sustained the family for some time and has coped well. But now he can let go and allow his rage and anger to come out.

The father has to adapt to changes in the mother as she gets well. "As she starts to feel better . . . she often begins to be more assertive in her relationship. She is able to ask clearly for what she needs and to say 'no' without being overwhelmed with guilt. Unfortunately, sometimes as she begins to feel stronger, her partner becomes distressed about the changes he sees in her and how they will affect him. Some couples choose to seek counseling to resolve these new conflicts," say experts from the Pacific Post Partum Support Society. When the wife is very dysfunctional, the husband can get psychologically distressed and may need support, too.

> *Postpartum Support International is what held me together. Jane [Honikman, founder of PSI] knew all about this illness. She gave me numbers of all these people to talk to.*

Even if the husband does not feel he needs individual therapy, he should recognize that feelings of resentfulness and irritability probably mean he is overextending himself. Fathers need to understand that it's very difficult to help someone when you are feeling negative. And your wife very much needs your help.

Husbands need to acknowledge their own need for support and to ask for it, say Robert and Susan Hickman. "Men take great pride in their ability to problem solve. Unfortunately, the added responsibilities they must assume are unfamiliar . . . Husbands may be unwilling to admit that they may be experiencing hardship or unable to articulate the need for support." But, they add, "clinical experience suggests that husbands are able to support their wives maximally when they feel support for their efforts."

This support cannot come from their wives. Instead, family members, friends, and health care professionals can help the father. It is enormously helpful if the husband's employer is understanding and supports his need to handle his problems at home.

The husband, or primary support person, should not neglect his own self-care. It's important for the father to adopt a "business as usual" attitude even though it's hard. He should try to see friends and do things he enjoys. He should ask for help when he needs it. The husband needs to remember to be hopeful; postpartum psychiatric illness is treatable and temporary. Remember that the patient is not the illness. The husband shouldn't take outbursts from the patient personally.

The husband needs to express what he feels. He can tell his wife when he can't be supportive or attentive by saying, "I love you and I'm trying to help you. But I can't deal with this right now." Likewise, he should tell his wife when he feels good and positive or sees good things about her recovery.

Support groups can be tremendously helpful to fathers. Fathers are invited to attend Depression After Delivery support groups, although few do, says DAD founder Nancy Berchtold. Fathers can call DAD to locate a telephone counselor, for example, another man who has dealt with postpartum illness. In a few places, postpartum support groups for men are available. Robert Hickman runs one such group in San Diego.

Support groups for fathers can help them reinterpret what is going on, Hickman says. For example, a father can learn that his wife's unresponsiveness is not a sign of personal rejection. Support groups can also help the husband know when to relinquish the child care responsibilities to his wife. Support groups help educate the husband about the medications his wife is taking and why she needs to take them for as long as her doctor instructs. In support groups, the husband can also learn about the risk of recurrence with future pregnancies. He can discover how other men in the group handled medical costs and battled their insurers for coverage. In short, Hickman says, "Husbands need to know that they are not the only ones going through this difficult set of circumstances."

THE INFANT AND CHILDREN

There is growing recognition that the father is forgotten in postpartum illness. However, another perspective comes from Dr. Edward Z. Tronick, chief of the Child Development Unit at Children's Hospital in Boston and a professor of pediatrics at Harvard Medical School: "We have made children the forgotten part. But, actually, the whole family is the forgotten part."

Women who suffer from postpartum blues or mild or short-lived postpartum depression need not fear that they have caused their children great or lasting harm. Children are resilient and survive our misfortunes and mistakes.

For women who suffer from serious and/or long-term illness, it is necessary to look at what effects the illness may have had on the infant and older children. The intent of this discussion is not to place guilt on the mother or deepen her despair over what this illness has cost her. Indeed, facing what effects the illness may have on her children might, in the long run, prevent the illness from doing more damage.

It is important, moreover, for the medical profession to remember that for every mother with a postpartum illness, there is at least one child who may be profoundly affected as well. Overall, thousands of children may be growing up under the care of a depressed mother and suffering the adverse effects. The rate of maternal depression — depressed mothers of young children — may be even higher than rates of postpartum depression. Tronick, who has done research on mother-child interaction and maternal depression, has tried to determine the rates of maternal depression by taking surveys at health centers where mothers bring their children for care. At Boston City Hospital, he found that 30 percent of mothers had symptoms of depression. The rate of depressive symptoms was 41 percent among mothers not living with fathers and 50 percent among mothers in non-English-speaking populations. The survey did not diagnose depression in these women; but it indicated, at the very least, the presence of minor depressions, "demoralizations that women are feeling at very high rates during the early years of their child-rearing experiences: sad, angry, helpless, sleep problems."[3]

What are the effects of a mother's sadness, anger, and fatigue on her child? The effects on children are not well studied. Separating the influence of heredity and environment is difficult. Moreover, there is great individuality in how children — even siblings — respond to a set of circumstances. The presence of other healthy, loving adults in a family can help offset negative consequences. And how the mother and her child or children work to re-establish their bonds soon after her recovery can also make a difference. In general, however, studies show children raised by depressed parents, especially mothers, are at high risk for delays in cognitive, social, and behavioral development.

EFFECTS ON INFANTS

I remember wanting my baby to disappear. I feared I might harm her so I avoided her. I think there were times when I left her alone in the crib and wandered aimlessly as if I were lost. I felt drawn back to my childhood and just wanted to be taken care of. I couldn't believe that this person that I wanted so much I now had no connection to.

The most valuable and surprising contributions to infant and child development in the 1990s are the findings on how a mother's behavior affects her baby. Obviously, an ill or confused mother may harbor negative emotions about childbirth and her baby. For example, depressed mothers are more likely to express negative or mixed feelings about their three-month-old babies, according to one study.[4] This finding was reinforced four years later, when another study also found that depressed mothers are more likely to express mixed feelings, indifference, or dislike for their three-month-old babies.[5]

But even when a mother holds strong feelings of love for her baby, the symptoms of the depression she is experiencing can affect the infant. A depressed mother's demeanor and behavior can subtly influence the mother-child relationship. Research shows an infant's relationship with its mother lays the foundation for its future personality and intellectual development. The foundation for this relationship begins in the first few weeks and months of life, when the mother is most likely to be acutely ill.

This tender period is critical to optimal child development, says Irving B. Harris, cofounder of the Ounce of Prevention Fund, a nonprofit organization dedicated to the welfare of children. "That is when the brain pathways that eventually lead to curiosity and empathy and trust begin to develop. That is when, in loving interaction with nurturing caregivers, babies learn that they can trust and feel loved and respected. That is when they begin to become human beings."

In a healthy mother-infant relationship, a smile is the primary form of attachment in an infant, says Dr. Bruce Taubman, author of *Curing Infant Colic.* "The first infant smiles, which occur in the second month, are spontaneous, but soon the baby begins to smile in response to the sight of a face. But that's only half of the story . . . the smile triggers an instinctive, genetically programmed set of behaviors in the mother — fondling, holding and talking."

Also, in the first three months the baby becomes secure that the environment is responsive to his or her cries. By four to six months of age, babies are aware that their mothers are responding to their communications. They can discriminate between different people and respond to their mothers differently from the way they respond to others, Taubman says. At seven or eight months of age, a baby will cry if a stranger approaches or the mother leaves the room.

This is the normal course of development. But if something goes wrong and the infant's signals are not met, the baby can fail to develop any attachment to a human being. This is what happened in a study of an English orphanage. Infants were cared for on a specific schedule but their attachment behaviors were ignored. The infants lost interest in eating, grew poorly, and showed retarded social behavior.

This is an extreme example. But, Taubman asks, what happens if the mother-infant attachment is somewhere in between? One study showed that mothers of infants who exhibited insecure infant-mother attachment:[6]

- Seemed inaccessible and insensitive to their infants
- Either failed to notice their infants' signals or, if they did notice, often ignored them
- Responded to their infants in ways that depended heavily on their own moods and activities
- Showed no understanding for their infants' individuality, but rather tried to impose their own will on the babies
- Became angry and resentful when the babies' behavior was irritating or annoying

According to Taubman, and other researchers, the key to a secure infant-parent relationship is the parents' responsiveness to the child. That means that early on, parents learn how to respond to the child. All parents feel they fail to respond appropriately at times, and "individual episodes of frustration and agitation will not permanently harm your baby any more than temporary frustration damages your own well-being." But when the frustration and agitation is long-lasting or chronic, the infant can start to suffer.

According to Tronick, "These little beings are designed to get resources from the environment. And most important are their communicative capacities. Everything from crying to smiling to facial expressiveness to gestures impact on their caregiver. The infant is dependent on caregivers to read those communicative signals and figure out what it is that the infant requires at this point in time, at this moment."

The simple interaction of a mother smiling and talking to her infant and eliciting smiles and coos from the baby is the beginning of the infant's development of social interaction skills. Moreover, the infant's cognitive abilities are influenced early on, too, because social interaction is an important cognitive task.

One study found that significant intellectual deficits were found in the children of mothers who had been depressed, but only when this depression had occurred in the first year.[7] Tronick found that at one year of age, infants of depressed mothers are less active and more distractible, express fewer positive emotions, cry more, are more angry, and exhibit less object and social engagement.

These studies suggested that the infants of depressed mothers also become depressed. In one study, by three months of age, infants of depressed mothers developed their own type of depressed behavior characterized by the lack of smiling and a tendency to look away from a face. Babies became more upset when they looked at their mother's unresponsive face than when they saw her leave the room. These babies develop a style of depressive interaction with all people, researchers found. It's even possible, one expert noted, that interaction with a depressed mother affects the development of apathy and withdrawal in a baby.[8]

The importance of having a secure base from which to explore the environment is paramount to an infant's development, says Tronick. "The child who can successfully form an attachment is a child who can then explore the world, is a child who can then move away from that secure base."

Baby boys may be more affected by a mother's depression than baby girls, research suggests. Mothers may even react differently depending on their baby's gender. One research project showed that depressed mothers acted more negatively with their sons, expressing more sadness and anger.

Although it's natural to wish that the infant has not been affected by a mother's depression, parents should persist — as should researchers — in trying to understand just how the baby's development may have been altered. Several studies are underway to explore that issue.

"I think the long-term follow-up of these children is going to be very exciting," says Dr. Lee Cohen, reproductive psychiatry expert at Massachusetts General Hospital and Harvard Medical School. "I think it will be one of the final pieces that allows us to put together a more refined formulation of how to limit maternal morbidity from postpartum psychiatric disorders."

CHILD ABUSE

A discussion of the effects of maternal depression is not complete or honest without discussing physical abuse. Studies show that from 23 to 56 percent of battered children are ten months to one year old when the act is first reported. Thus, much child abuse could begin in the postpartum period. Most likely, for those who abuse their infants, postpartum depression is not the only cause. These mothers may also have a greater risk for abusing. For example, they themselves may have been abused as children.

The risk of infanticide among women with postpartum psychosis is well known. But it is simply not known whether the symptoms of postpartum depression alone increase the risk of child abuse. However, one found study that depressed parents were twice as likely to become frustrated with their children, and were almost twice as likely to yell at or spank them.[9] And, mothers with postpartum depression sometimes became emotionally volatile with babies during the first six months, according to another study.[10] These babies were often withdrawn and did not look directly at their mothers.

The repercussions of child abuse are often serious and long lasting. This may be even more true if the abusive parent was also depressed or mentally ill at the time. One study of abused elementary school children found that those who had depressed mothers also had the most serious behavior problems.[11]

EFFECTS ON CHILDREN

My son had low priority. It was up to relatives to take care of him. I felt the best thing for me and him was to get his mother back in shape.

Most research suggests that babies six months to eighteen months old are the most vulnerable for enduring the effects of a mother's depression. Studies are conflicting regarding the effects of maternal depression in children and whether maternal depression in the postpartum period is reflected in children later, at preschool age or older. One report, however, found that depressed parents reacted and behaved less positively with their children than non-depressed parents. The depressed parents were less likely to read to their children, sing or play music with them, or hug or cuddle them, and they even engaged in fewer routines, such as fixing meals and giving the children baths.[12]

In general, research shows that preschool children of depressed parents exhibit a higher level of emotionality. An increased incidence of headaches, stomachaches, and accidents are also reported in these children.

The length of time the mother is depressed undoubtedly plays a role in the effects on the children. The children of women with postpartum illness who have many recurrences of depression or who have a long-lasting initial bout of illness have a higher risk of suffering.

Generally, studies show that school-age children with one or more depressed parents have more acting out. Preschool children have problems with selective attention and frustration, and exhibit less prosocial behavior. One study found that children of the same sex as the depressed parent were more likely to suffer.[13]

Having a depressed parent can increase the risk that the child, too, will develop depression. Studies show childhood depression has both physiological and environmental causes. One study showed that a child whose mother is depressed has a 30 percent chance of showing signs of depression by age six or seven; a 50 percent chance if both parents have depression.[14] Depressed children lag academically and become socially withdrawn and isolated. Research also shows that these children demonstrate excessive rivalry and fighting with siblings and are impatient and withdrawn.

In older children, depressed mothers are more likely to threaten punishment and not go through with it or to forget promises, experts suggest. They are less likely to encourage achievement. This could be due to the mother's feelings of helplessness, a preoccupation with herself, or decreased memory.

Families with depressed mothers have increased conflict and decreased expressiveness, cohesion, and organization. Marital discord is also common in these families and can contribute to child behavior problems. "Thus, depression in a mother has a direct effect on her children via her own behaviors . . . and an indirect effect via family dysfunction," noted one author. But, children can be protected by having a good relationship with one healthy parent or grandparent.

> *My psychiatrist told me that as long as my son had warm, loving care, it doesn't need to come from me. My mother and mother-in-law took care of him and I took care of myself. I didn't have a lot of guilt about that. And now I'm very close to my son.*

Moreover, some depressed women are able to communicate warmly and responsively to their young children. And the length of the mother's depression is a major factor on the effects on children. "It would be less worrying if the depression were transient, but it is persistent and is associated with behavioral, developmental, or emotional problems of children," say pediatricians Barry S. Zuckerman and William R. Beardslee, Boston-based experts in behavioral pediatrics, who have written on maternal depression.

Children may feel responsible for their mother's symptoms of anger, withdrawal, and sadness. At times, children may even be accused — either directly or indirectly — of being responsible for it. "Children need to understand that their mother has an illness and that, although all children do 'bad' things sometimes, the children are not responsible for their mothers' illnesses," Zuckerman and Beardslee say.

Therapy is highly successful in helping children cope with the effects of depression in the family. This therapy can begin for older children while the mother herself is in therapy. Or the repercussions on the children can be addressed later, when the mother has recovered, without long-term or dire consequences to the family. Families need only to remember that the effects on the children should be considered and parents should not hesitate to obtain professional counseling for their children. Children of mothers with long-term or chronic depression should be watched for learning and behavior problems as well as affective disorders.

Women with postpartum psychiatric illness should not be blamed for the effects of their illness in their children. Neither should a women who suffered a postpartum illness and recovered and whose child later developed behavioral or cognitive problems be blamed as the cause of her child's problems.

Remember that major illnesses — cancer, heart disease, depression — commonly affect the family as well as the patient. Everyone feels the strain. However, families that stay together, love one another, share their concerns and feelings openly, and bury the urge to blame someone or something will end up valuing and respecting each other more, not less.

CHAPTER TEN

Recurrence and Prevention

I had postpartum depression with my first child eleven years ago. No one talked about postpartum depression then, and I just mumbled through it. I wasn't prepared for it to happen again.

Many women claim that they wish their doctor or nurse practitioner or childbirth educator or mother had warned them of the possibility that they might suffer from a postpartum disorder. But if the risk of a postpartum disorder were discussed before childbirth, would that be enough to prevent the illness?

That question has many answers. Some experts suggest that women who suffer postpartum disorders that are largely due to psychosocial issues — such as having too high expectations of themselves as mothers and trying to do too much — might be able to bypass the illness if they were better educated and informed about the psychosocial factors that lead to postpartum disorders.[1] Others contend that even postpartum blues — thought to be hormonally based — might be less disruptive and severe if women were encouraged to talk about the blues and ask questions before childbirth. Moreover, if their husbands were informed of the blues they might be better able to recognize it and help their wives.[2]

Women who suffer from postpartum depression, postpartum psychosis, or an anxiety disorder have illnesses that are more difficult to prevent. But there are several important exceptions:

- Early recognition and treatment can drastically alter the course of postpartum depression, psychosis, or anxiety.
- Some women have obvious risk factors that can alert physicians to the possibility of a postpartum disorder (such as women who have a past history of mental illness). Women with a high-risk profile should be treated cautiously during pregnancy, birth, and the postpartum period.
- Women who suffered a previous postpartum disorder are at high risk for a recurrence and should be aware of the many alternatives available to avoid another illness.

PREVENTION FOR ALL NEW MOTHERS

Postpartum experts agree that many cases of illness could be prevented or significantly altered if a woman's mental health status during and after pregnancy was given greater consideration by health professionals. Prevention can take place at prenatal visits, the six-week postpartum visit, prepared childbirth classes, and pediatrician visits.

"Are we doing all we should to prevent those illnesses from occurring?" asks Dr. Deborah Sharp, a London-based obstetrician. "I believe that we are not and that our preventive role begins during pregnancy, when women are receiving such intensive medical care."

During pregnancy, simple questions can be asked of a woman regarding her prior psychiatric history, family psychiatric history, ambivalence about pregnancy, relationship with the baby's father, relationship with her own mother, role models, support, recent losses and/or stressors, and prior pregnancy loss, says Dr. Christa Hines, a St. Louis, Missouri, postpartum expert. But, says Sharp: "How often is a woman given time to talk about these personal and sometimes distressing feelings during her appointment?"

Asking pregnant patients questions regarding financial problems, problems in previous pregnancies, specific fears about labor and delivery, past psychiatric history, and social support increases the detection rate of postpartum disorders by 25 percent, Sharp suggests. If the physician asked the mother to complete a general health questionnaire, that could help increase the detection rate by another 25 percent, Sharp says.

Most of the emphasis on prevention during the prenatal period should focus on psychosocial factors that will help new parents with the adjustment to parenthood. This would benefit all couples regardless of whether the woman develops a postpartum illness. "Many studies show that prenatal psychosocial interventions can significantly help in the successful adjustment to the parental role, and thereby counteract the development of postpartum depression," says Dr. Elizabeth Herz, a postpartum expert in Washington, D.C.

In one study in which new mothers were given general education about caring for a new baby, researchers found that informed mothers had greater success caring for their babies, and that their babies were less irritable, slept better, and were easier to feed.[3] This study is evidence of the power of preparation and education. Preparation could include lowering the mother's expectations and dispelling the myths surrounding motherhood, strengthening marital support, reducing outside stress factors, rearranging priorities, and encouraging the mother to get help and advice in regard to her infant.

Says Herz: "Ideally, this preventive mental health intervention would be undertaken by the obstetrician as part of the prenatal care for the high-risk patient."

Pregnant women need to be reassured of their fears but also cautioned that things may not turn out as they envision. "We need to reassure them that what's going to happen is, hopefully, what they expect but to keep their goals reasonable," says Dr. Tamara Ostapowicz, an obstetrician from St. Louis, Missouri. "I think the women who come in with the highest expectations are sometimes let down and depressed if they don't work exactly . . . And the patients who come in with their four-page list of what they want to see happen, if they get 50%, that's lucky."

Parents should be told that they will receive conflicting advice about babies and that they need to lower their expectations, Ostapowicz says. "I tell my patients to try to get two things done [after they bring the baby home] and if they get one done, that's 50% and that's not bad. A lot of them need permission from the physician to do that . . . They'll do it if it comes from the health care provider."

In addition to benefiting from the obstetrician's efforts at prevention, a great many couples participate in prepared childbirth classes, where they learn about the risk of postpartum illness. Childbirth classes are the most successful method of getting the father involved in the pregnancy and, thus, could set him up as an ally if things go wrong after childbirth. These groups also help parents to meet other parents, and some mothers remain in touch after childbirth and even begin new mother groups.

All childbirth educators should have enough training and knowledge to explain the risk factors and symptoms of postpartum disorders and to inform parents of how to seek help. Although there is much to learn in childbirth classes, even a few minutes devoted to the end of the final session might be enough to persuade a new parent to get help when things begin to go wrong at home. Childbirth educators have sometimes resisted including postpartum mental health issues in their courses because, they claim, prospective new parents are too concerned with the immediate issues — getting through childbirth — to listen to what might happen after bringing the baby home. Some childbirth educators also say that prospective parents don't want to believe anything bad — like a postpartum illness — might happen to them and, thus, tune out that kind of information.

Although these objections might be valid to some extent, childbirth educators should not shirk or dismiss this convenient opportunity to help parents prevent what could be a tragic situation. One childbirth educator said she impressed upon her classes the importance of recognizing a postpartum depression by adopting a serious tone and speaking intently for just a few minutes about the need to be aware of changes in a new mother's personality and when to call for help. She made a point of alerting fathers that this responsibility falls on their shoulders.

Other childbirth educators merely include a pamphlet or brochure about postpartum illness in the stack of educational materials that is given to couples in classes. These pamphlets are often provided by local support groups for postpartum depression or local hospitals or health professionals who offer postpartum care.

In general, new parents only need to be given some simple postpartum advice, Seattle-based postpartum expert Dawn Gruen says. This includes:

- Know the basic symptoms of postpartum illness and how to call someone if several symptoms are present for more than three weeks.
- Make sure the person you call knows about postpartum disorders.
- Make sure the new mother gets plenty of rest.
- Ask for help.
- Lower your expectations.
- Don't deny your feelings.
- Don't feel guilty about how you are feeling.
- Locate the stressors in your life and remove them.

"It is imperative for all childbirth educators to be knowledgeable and informed about the risk factors, symptoms, treatment, and prevention of postpartum depression," says DAD founder Nancy Berchtold.

"Warm lines" — telephone counseling services — which are usually sponsored by hospitals, provide new parents with opportunities for recognizing postpartum illness. They can also provide information about new parent support groups located in community education centers or pediatricians' offices.

The obstetrician has two additional opportunities to warn the new parents of the possibility of postpartum illness: at discharge from the hospital and at the six-week postpartum exam. At the six-week checkup, the physician could ask such questions as How are things going at home with the baby? How are you sleeping and eating? and Is your energy level good?

Although women with a history of mental illness have a much higher risk of suffering a postpartum psychiatric illness, it is the women who become ill "out of the blue" who oftentimes represent the most tragic cases. "I worry about the low-risk patient," says Dr. Lee Cohen, expert in reproductive psychiatry at Massachusetts General Hospital and Harvard Medical School. "We don't do a good job of screening in obstetrics or pediatrics. And it's a tragedy that these women present [for psychiatric treatment] at six or nine months out who are extremely ill."

PREVENTING A RECURRENCE OF POSTPARTUM ILLNESS

Almost every woman and her spouse who undergo a serious postpartum illness ask if they dare undertake another pregnancy. Will it happen again? Could it be even worse the second time? Is there any way to prevent it?

The truth is that there is overwhelming evidence that women who have had a postpartum disorder are at high risk of experiencing a similar illness with subsequent pregnancies. According to Cohen, the risk of relapse is as follows:

Previous illness	Chance of relapse
Postpartum Psychosis	75% – 90%
Postpartum Depression	50%
Bipolar Disorder	50%
Major Depression	30%

"Sometimes the second illness was worse than the first, and in others it was of the same severity or not quite so bad, but in every case it was bad enough to require further medical treatment," says Dr. Katharina Dalton in her book *Depression After Childbirth.* According to Dr. Ricardo Fernandez, assistant professor of clinical psychology at the Robert Woods Johnson/Rutgers Medical School, many women who have recurrences experience the same type of illness as the first time. Yet, not every woman has a recurrence. And, Dalton notes, "there seemed to be no way in which a recurrence could be predicted."

PROPHYLAXIS

Most experts feel that a woman who has had a postpartum illness and wants a second child should have one because (1) the risks of suffering a recurrence can be minimized and (2) the illness can be anticipated and treated successfully. Many women who take preventive measures and undergo a second pregnancy are relieved with the outcome.

> *To know, the second time, that people really understood what was happening to us made the birth and being a mom everything I always dreamed it would be and more when I had my son, as opposed to the first time.*

But, having a second child often means submitting to more monitoring by health professionals (more appointments, more phone calls, more questions). The woman and her spouse should be willing to face the risk and should prepare to do things differently the second time. For example, some women require medication immediately after childbirth to prevent the onset of depression or psychosis and, therefore, must be willing to forego breastfeeding.

According to Fernandez, there are two ways to reduce recurrence: the psychosocial approach and the biological approach. The psychosocial interventions can begin as soon as the woman learns she is pregnant. They include setting up a good, strong, and large support system at home so that the mother can rest and be relieved of outside stressors; making arrangements for caring for the older children and even the infant, if necessary; and reviewing the things the mother can do to reduce symptoms, such as eating well and resting.

Educational preparation can include planning free time, arranging for use of a babysitter, and developing a support system, say experts with the Pacific Post Partum Support Society. In addition, the couple should examine their beliefs and expectations about their second child and should be flexible regarding their birth plan. And the mother should postpone decisions about her career.

I know, next time, to get help. I'm also learning healthy things that will help me. Breastfeeding was really hard for me. The next baby will use a bottle.

"When I work with moms . . . who are trying to prevent a recurrence, I'll see them at certain times during their pregnancy to make sure that a lot of these things are already set ahead of time," Fernandez says. There is a tendency for couples who have endured a postpartum illness to deny that it will happen again and to ignore the risk.

I'm having a new baby, and it's amazing how [the experience] starts to fade out. I don't even want to think about it. But I sat down the other day and reviewed notes and articles I had about the illness. It brought it all back.

"Sometimes one of the problems with moms who have postpartum disorders is that as soon as they get better, they kind of go away and they never want to hear about the illness again,"

Fernandez says. "They go back into the denial that if they have another child they are not going to have a recurrence. The problem with that is, if you're not aware of it or you tend to deny it you tend to let the symptoms [go for a longer period of time]."

Ideally, couples who have experienced a postpartum disorder should discuss their plans for pregnancy with their physician before conception. Women in therapy should also discuss their feelings about a second pregnancy.

"If you still have a lot of painful feelings and memories left from your previous experience, it may be a good idea to look for some counseling to help you sort them out," say experts with the Pacific Post Partum Support Society. "Do not be afraid or ashamed to ask for this help, if you can. You will be able to cope much better with successive births."

Couples should discuss when and how to tell other people about the second pregnancy and should be prepared for intrusive, even insensitive remarks. Some relatives might ask why the couple would want to risk it again. Others might suggest that the illness won't happen again. Couples should plan their response to these remarks and hold fast to their own plans and beliefs regarding the pregnancy.

Everyone says it won't happen again because now you know how to take care of a baby. No one understands.

THE BIOLOGICAL APPROACH TO PREVENTION

Women who are still undergoing medical treatment for their previous postpartum illness often need to go off medications before getting pregnant. Lithium, for example, can produce birth defects in 10 percent of all pregnancies. Lithium treatment can sometimes be restored in the final month of pregnancy. Decisions on medications taken during pregnancy must be made with a careful consideration of the possible benefits versus the possible health risks to the baby, says Dr. Lori Altshuler, a Los Angeles psychiatrist with expertise in treatment of mental disorders during pregnancy.

No drug is approved by the U.S. Food and Drug Administration for use during pregnancy, and all psychotropic medications cross the placenta and can impact the growing fetus. On the other hand, Altshuler notes, "because a growing number of studies demonstrate high rates of relapse when medications are discontinued in patients suffering from mood disorders, anxiety disorders, and schizophrenia, the decision to stop pharmacologic treatment when women with these disorders become pregnant or plan to conceive becomes that much more difficult."

In general, research has shown tricyclic antidepressants to be relatively safe when taken during pregnancy. Likewise, early studies of Prozac used in pregnancy also appear to be safe for the fetus. Lithium, however, has proved problematic, especially when taken in the first trimester. Moreover, because of the metabolic demands of the body during pregnancy, higher doses may be required of any medications given at that time compared with nonpregnant periods.

If medication is administered, attempts should be made to use the lowest dose possible, Altshuler says. A decision on what course to pursue is "complex and delicate." Although it's important to prevent recurring mental illness, the mother's self-esteem may also be tied to the sense of not causing her fetus any harm.

Once the woman is pregnant and the psychosocial preparations have begun, the couple should discuss the use of prophylactic medications with the physician. The use of medications to prevent a recurrence of postpartum illness is controversial because there are few good studies that show if prophylaxis really works, says Herz. Prophylaxis in the postpartum period can include estrogen, thyroid medications, lithium, and antidepressants.

The most conservative approach to preventing a recurrence is to do nothing but watch the mother very closely. This might be a suitable option for a woman who suffered a very mild depression or who can identify psychosocial risk factors that might have contributed to her first illness but which have been eliminated in her life since.

The next approach would be to administer hormones to the mother immediately after childbirth in the attempt to offset the drop in hormones that is thought to contribute to postpartum illness. Progesterone is one such therapy, but its use is controversial because there are reports of women becoming even worse on the therapy. Another hormonal therapy is progesterone with estrogen. This approach aims to bolster both hormones that are known to plunge following childbirth. However, it has more side effects. Estrogen stops milk production. And estrogen is linked to long-term side effects like breast cancer. Other studies have tested estrogen alone and estrogen with antidepressants.

Thyroid medication is another possibility. It can also be administered to women who show low thyroid levels after childbirth.

Finally, women can receive antidepressants or antipsychotic drugs to prevent a recurrence. A woman who suffered depression could be given the same antidepressant that helped her the first time. Drug therapy could begin around the same time as her previous illness began; for example, one-week postpartum or one-month postpartum. Psychotic women who were helped by lithium the first time might be given lithium again immediately after delivery. The antipsychotic drugs can be given in low doses prophylactically.

Women should carefully select their health care providers during a second pregnancy. Was the obstetrician competent in handling the postpartum disorder the first time? Is the obstetrician willing to work with other health professionals, such as a psychiatrist, during the second pregnancy? It's frightening to go through pregnancy and childbirth after having suffered a postpartum illness, and confidence in health care providers is essential.

My doctor suggested I take estrogen this time after the birth. I hope I'm in good hands.

The story of Donna is a typical example of a woman who did all the right things in her second pregnancy, with great success:

Donna was twenty-six and her husband was thirty when they married. She worked as a nurse in an operating room. He owned a business. They were happily married and planned on having a family soon after marriage. They had been married for two years when Donna became pregnant. The pregnancy was an easy one. Donna worked until ten days before her due date. The couple then moved to a new house and Donna spent the next two weeks readying the nursery.

Ten days past her due date, Donna went into labor. The labor was treacherous, lasting thirty-nine hours and requiring the use of several medications. Donna pushed for three hours before the baby boy was born with the help of forceps.

"I wanted it to be natural, but it didn't work out that way," she said.

The baby was healthy and the couple rejoiced. But the brightness began to fade quickly for Donna. She suffered headaches and didn't sleep during the three days she was in the hospital.

"I felt a change, but I really didn't realize the extent. I would just sort of lay there thinking about things."

At home, Donna felt alone and isolated in her upstairs bedroom while breastfeeding her son. When her mother called to ask if she could help, Donna would refuse. "You just have this idea that you can do it all yourself."

But the tough labor had taken its toll on the young mother. Donna became constipated and had pain and bleeding when moving her bowels. Once, she had to go to an emergency room for bleeding. She was prescribed enemas and had to remain in bed at home. She was exhausted. She still couldn't sleep. Her personality rapidly changed.

"My family knew I just wasn't myself. I just felt I couldn't sleep. I had rapid speech and was repeating thoughts."

Finally, an argument with her husband and advice from a friend convinced Donna she needed help. She went to a hospital to talk to someone. But, to her dismay, she was kept there while her family was summoned. Doctors told Donna that she was psychotic.

Donna was admitted to a hospital inpatient psychiatric program and remained there for thirty days. There, she learned she had a postpartum disorder. She began treatment with lithium and improved. After her discharge, she continued with psychiatric outpatient treatment. Donna's depression lingered for about two years — an unusually long course — and she continued taking medications. She decided not to go back to work. Instead, she went back to school, became involved in her church, and taught Sunday school.

She also learned about Depression After Delivery and began educating herself about postpartum illness. She said, "It was like a light went on."

When her son was three, Donna's birth control failed and she became pregnant again. "I always wanted to have more children, but I wanted to do it feeling secure with a physician and obstetrician to help me. I was in a panic."

She changed to a new obstetrics group comprised of two male doctors and one female doctor. The male doctors told Donna not to worry about her previous illness. However, the female doctor, upon hearing about Donna's illness, referred her to a local specialist in postpartum disorders. Donna was lucky to live in a city with a hospital renowned for its treatment of postpartum illness.

When she was five months pregnant, Donna and her husband went to see the postpartum expert. The expert told Donna her chances of experiencing a recurrence was 66 percent. The expert sent letters to Donna's obstetricians to alert them of Donna's risk and to convince them to treat her with special care. The postpartum expert also presented Donna and her husband with three choices. Donna could go on lithium (the drug that helped her the first time) after the birth. Or she could start another antipsychotic drug that might allow Donna to continue to breastfeed as long as she and the baby underwent blood tests. Or she could do nothing and wait to see if symptoms developed.

"My husband said, 'Donna, chances are so high.' So we decided to go with the lithium because I knew it worked for me before. I felt breastfeeding wasn't that important."

The couple's daughter was born normally after only three hours of labor. "It was a totally different experience. Things just really fell into place," Donna said.

Donna remained on lithium for about four months then eased off the drug. "I felt I had already taken the right steps. I had the doctor to fall back on. I felt good with the doctor. I also knew during the second pregnancy not to make major changes. I found out about a support group for postpartum disorders. I started to attend meetings and that was very helpful to me. I had people around me who knew about the illness. It's such a big help to have other people to talk to. Normal moms really don't understand."

When Mental Illness Recurs After a Postpartum Illness

Many health professionals assume that a woman who suffers a postpartum disorder will not necessarily be prone to other mental health disorders, unrelated to childbirth, later in life. This is probably assumed because postpartum disorders are thought to be highly influenced by rapidly changing hormones — something that happens only after childbirth. Moreover, because many women who have postpartum disorders have had no prior history of mental illness, there would be little reason to assume they would be at high risk again, except after pregnancy.

But there is little support for these assumptions. And, in fact, there is little known about the risk of recurrence of mental health problems for these women outside of childbirth events. Research on women and depression in general shows that they are highly susceptible to repeated bouts of the illness, especially if they are untreated, under-treated, or inadequately treated.

Moreover, depression in women is an illness that should be viewed in relation to a woman's changing hormonal makeup over the entire life cycle, say Ellen McGrath, Gwendolyn Puryear Keita, Bonnie Strickland, and Nancy Felipe Russo, the authors of *Women and Depression.* "A life cycle perspective appears to be one of the keys to understanding depression in women," they say.

Experts differ on whether women who suffer from postpartum disorders will continue to be at high risk for later mental health problems. Fernandez has seen only two women with continuing psychiatric problems. "What my experience suggests is that if you have a postpartum disorder, it means that, as a woman, you are susceptible to psychiatric problems around any hormonal event."

This can include mood disorders around the time of menstruation or menopause.

Research on depression in general, however, suggests that the brain can become sensitive to bouts of depression no matter what caused the initial episode. This research on brain chemistry and depression, however, is very new, and no one really understands all the factors involved in the emergence of mental health problems.

Perhaps the most significant point for you to remember is that you might be at higher risk for continuing mental health problems. This does not imply that you or your family need to worry about the future; only that you should be aware of the signs and symptoms of illness and who you can contact for help. It is important for you to explore the tendency to deny that you might ever be ill again. Remember that early recognition and early treatment can nip in the bud many mental illnesses and dramatically reduce any potential repercussions.

> *There are still times I feel "fragile" and lack the confidence I once had. Over the years I began to process what happened to me with the support of a caring husband and family.*

It is also useful to keep in mind these risk factors that are linked to the recurrence of mental disorders in general:

1. Being overly preoccupied with work (for example, working very long hours)
2. Having no time or energy for the family
3. Having no time to enjoy outside interests, or to exercise or play
4. Eating poorly
5. Being irritable and less sensitive of others
6. Holding back feelings instead of expressing them

Women who experience a postpartum disorder shouldn't be afraid to embrace life and live it to its fullest. Having a beautiful child to raise and to love requires that kind of commitment along with the expectation that life is good and things will be okay. But it's also appropriate to reserve a tiny part of your mind for the memories of a difficult time. Being vigilant means you hold your own best interests at heart.

Woman must not accept; she must challenge. She must not be awed by that which has been built up around her; she must reverence that woman in her which struggles for expression.

— Margaret Sanger

Resources

Postpartum Organizations

Depression After Delivery
PO Box 1282, Morrisville, PA 19067
800-944-4PPD
(A self-help, mutual-aid support group. Refers calls to local support groups throughout the United States. Provides telephone counselors.)

Postpartum Support International
927 N. Kellogg Ave., Santa Barbara, CA 93111
805-967-7636
(An organization for consumers and professionals interested in advancing knowledge about postpartum disorders and treatment. Refers calls to local support groups and professionals. Operates a lending library. Hosts annual conferences on postpartum illness.)

Mother Care Services

The National Association of Postpartum Care Services
800-45-DOULA

Mothers Matter
171 Wood St., Rutherford, NJ 07070
201-933-8191
(Supports mothers in their parenting efforts.)

National Association of Mothers' Centers
336 Fulton Ave., Hempstead, NY 11550
516-486-6614

Mental Illness

National Alliance for the Mentally Ill
2101 Wilson Blvd., Suite 302, Arlington, VA 22201
703-524-7600

National Mental Health Association
1021 Prince St., Alexandria, VA 22314-2971
800-969-NMHA
(http://www.worldcorp.com.dc-online/nmha)

Depression

National Depressive and Manic Depressive Association
730 North Franklin St., Suite 501, Chicago, IL 60610
800-82-NDMDA

D/ART (Depression/Awareness, Recognition, and Treatment)
Write: Public Inquiries
National Institute of Mental Health
5600 Fishers Lane, Room 15-C-05, Rockville, MD 20807
800-421-4211

National Foundation for Depressive Illness
PO Box 2257, New York, NY 10116
800-248-4344

National Alliance for Research on Schizophrenia and Depression
60 Cutter Mill Road, Suite 200, Great Neck, NY, 11021
516-829-0091
(http://www.mhsource.com./narsad.html)

Obsessive-Compulsive Disorder

OCD Foundation, Inc.
PO Box 70, Milford, CT 60460-0070
203-874-3843

Anxiety

Anxiety Disorders Association of America
600 Executive Blvd., Suite 513, Rockville, MD 20852
301-231-9350
(http:/www.users.interport.net/~lindy/adaa.html)

Addiction

Alcoholics Anonymous
PO Box 459, Grant Central Station, New York, NY 10163
212-870-3400

National Association for Perinatal Addiction Research and
Education
200 N. Michigan Ave., Suite 300, Chicago, IL 60601
312-541-1272

Child Abuse

Parents Anonymous
675 W. Foothill Blvd., Suite 220, Claremont, CA 91711
909-621-6184
(Helps parents who are abusing their children or who are at high
risk for abusing their children.)

National Child Abuse Hotline
Childhelp USA
IOF Foresters
1345 El Centro Ave., PO Box 630, Hollywood, CA 90028
800-4ACHILD

National Committee to Prevent Child Abuse
332 S. Michigan Ave., Suite 1600, Chicago, IL 60604
800-CHILDREN (244-5373)

National Council on Child Abuse and Family Violence
1155 Connecticut Ave., N.W., #400, Washington, DC 20036
800-222-2000

Mothers' Special Services

Single Mothers By Choice
PO Box 1642, Gracie Square Station, New York, NY 10028
212-988-0993

Mothers At Home
8310-A Old Courthouse Road, Vienna, VA 22180
703-827-5903
(Supports mothers who remain at home to care for their children.)

Parents Without Partners
8807 Colesville Road, Silver Spring, MD 20910
301-588-9354

La Leche League International
1400 North Meacham Rd.
Schaumburg, IL 60173
847-519-7730

Grief Support

The Compassionate Friends
PO Box 3696, Oak Brook, IL 60522-3696
708-990-0010

Pregnancy and Infant Loss Center
1421 E. Wayzata Blvd., No. 30, Wayzata, MN 55391
612-473-9372

Share-Pregnancy and Infant Loss Support
St. Joseph's Health Center, 300 1st Capitol Dr.,
St. Charles, MO 63301
314-947-6164

Violence

National Coalition Against Domestic Violence
PO Box 18749, Denver, CO 80218
303-839-1852

VOICES in Action, Inc.
(Victims of Incest Can Emerge Survivors in Action)
PO Box 148309, Chicago, IL 60614
312-327-1500

National Victim Center
2111 Wilson Blvd., Suite 300, Arlington, VA 22201
703-276-2880
(http://www.nvc.org)

National Clearinghouse on Marital and Date Rape
2325 Oak St., Berkeley, CA 94708
510-524-1582

Infertility

American Society for Reproductive Medicine
1209 Montgomery Hwy., Birmingham, AL 35216
205-578-5000

Resolve
1310 Broadway, Somerville, MA 02144-1731
617-623-1156 or 617-623-0744
(Support organization for couples affected by infertility.)

Therapy

American Association for Marriage and Family Therapy
1133 15th St., N.W., Suite 300, Washington, DC 20005-2710
202-452-0109
(http://www.aamft.org)

American Psychiatric Association
1400 K St., N.W., Washington, DC 20005
202-682-6325
(http://www.thebody.com/apa/apapage.html)

American Psychological Association
1200 17th St., N.W., Washington, DC 20002
202-336-5500
(PsychNET-http://www.apa.org)

National Association of Social Workers
750 1st St. N.E., Suite 700, Washington, DC 20002
800-638-8799

American Mental Health Counselors Association
5999 Stevenson Ave., Alexandria, VA 22304
703-823-9800

Women of Color

National Latina Health Organization
PO Box 7567, Oakland, CA 94601
510-534-1362

National Black Women's Health Project
1237 Ralph David Abernathy Blvd., S.W., Atlanta, GA 30310
404-758-9590

National Asian Women's Health Organization
250 Montgomery St., Suite 410, San Francisco, CA 94140
415-989-9747

RECOMMENDED READING

Berg, B., *The Crisis of the Working Mother*, Summit Books, New York, 1986.

Brockington, I.F., Kumar, R., *Motherhood and Mental Illness*, Academic Press, London. Grune & Stratton, New York, 1982.

Fischer, L. *Linked Lives: Adult Daughters and Their Mothers*, Harper & Row, New York, 1986.

Gilligan, C., *In a Different Voice: Psychological Theory and Women's Development*, Harvard University Press, Cambridge, 1982.

Greenberg, M., *The Birth of a Father*, Avon Books, New York, 1985.

Hamilton, J., Harberger, P.N., *Postpartum Psychiatric Illness: A Picture Puzzle*, University of Pennsylvania Press, Philadelphia, 1992.

Jordan, J.; Kaplan, A.; Miller, J.M.; Stiver, I.; Surrey, J., *Women's Growth in Connection*, Guilford Press, New York, 1991.

Kitzinger, S., *Women as Mothers*, Martin Robinson Co. Ltd., London, 1978.

Kumar, R.; Brockington, I.F., *Motherhood and Mental Illness 2: Causes and Consequences*, Wright, London, 1988.

McGrath, E.; Keita, G.P.; Strickland, B.; Russo, N.F., *Women and Depression*, American Psychological Association, Washington, DC, 1990.

Miller, J.B., *Toward a New Psychology of Women*, Beacon Press, Boston, 1976.

Pacific Post Partum Support Society, "Post Partum Depression and Anxiety," Vancouver, BC, 1987.

Price, J., *Motherhood: What It Does to Your Mind*, Pandora, London, 1989.

Swigart, J., *The Myth of the Bad Mother*, Doubleday, New York, 1991.

For Children

Laskin, P.; Moskowitz, A., *Wish Upon a Star: A Story for Children with a Parent Who Is Mentally Ill*, Bunner-Mazel, New York, 1991.

Bibliography

Altshuler, L. et al., "Pharmacologic Management of Psychiatric Illness During Pregnancy: Dilemmas and Guidelines," *American Journal of Psychiatry, Vol. 153,* No. 5, May 1996.

Arboleda-Florez, J., "Infanticide: Some Medicolegal Considerations," *Canadian Psychiatric Association Journal, Vol. 20,* 1975.

Asch, S.; Rubin, L., "Postpartum Reactions: Some Unrecognized Variations," *American Journal of Psychiatry, Vol. 131,* No. 8, August 1974.

Atkinson, L.S. et al., "Postpartum Fatigue," *American Family Physician,* Vol. 50, No. 1, July 1994.

Beattie, J., "Observations on Post-Natal Depression, and a Suggestion for Its Prevention," *International Journal of Social Psychiatry,* Vol. 4, No. 4, Winter 1978.

Beck, C. Tatano, "The Effects of Postpartum Depression on Maternal-Infant Interaction: A Meta-analysis," *Nursing Research,* Sept./Oct. 1995.

Berchtold, N., "Depression After Delivery — Help from the Childbirth Educator," *International Journal of Childbirth Educators,* August 1978.

Berchtold, N.; Burrough, M., "Reaching Out: Depression After Delivery Support Group Network. *NAACOG'S Perinatal and Women's Health Nursing,* Vol. 1, No. 3.

Berg, B., *The Crisis of the Working Mother,* Summit Books, New York, 1986.

Bernstein, J. et al., "Effect of Previous Infertility on Maternal-Fetal Attachment, Coping Styles, and Self-Concept During Pregnancy," *Journal of Women's Health*, Vol. 3, No. 2, 1994.

Bower, B., "A Melancholy Breach: Science and Clinical Tradition Clash Amid New Insights Into Depression," *Science News*, No. 139, Jan. 26, 1991.

Brockington, I.F., "Maternity Blues and Post-Partum Euphoria," *British Journal of Psychiatry*, Vol. 152, 433-34, 1986.

Brockington, I.F. et al., "Puerperal Psychosis: Phenomena and Diagnosis," *Archives of General Psychiatry*, Vol. 38, July 1981.

Brody, J., "Beyond Tender Loving Care, Nurses Are a Force in Research," *New York Times*, Aug. 13, 1991.

The Bureau of National Affairs, Inc., *BNA Criminal Practice Manual*, Vol. 2, No. 21, Oct. 19, 1988.

Carnegie Corp., "A Decent Start: Promoting Healthy Child Development in the First Three Years of Life," New York, 1990.

Chodorow, N., *The Reproduction of Mothering*, University of California Press, Berkeley, 1978.

Cogill, S.R. et al., "Impact of Maternal Postnatal Depression on Cognitive Development of Young Children," *British Medical Journal*, Vol. 292, May 3, 1986.

Cole, K.C., *What Only a Mother Can Tell You About Having a Baby*, Berkeley, New York, 1981.

The Commonwealth Fund Survey of Parents with Young Children, The Commonwealth Fund, New York, Aug. 1996.

Consumer Reports, "Mental Health: Does Therapy Help?" Nov. 1995.

Cooper, P. et al., "Non-Psychotic Psychiatric Disorder After Childbirth: A Prospective Study of Prevalence, Incidence, Course and Nature," *British Journal of Psychiatry*, Vol. 252, 799-806, 1988.

Cox, J.L.; Holtden, J.M.; Sagovsky, R., "Detection of Postnatal Depression: Development of the 10-Item Edinburgh Postnatal Scale," *British Journal of Psychiatry*, Vol. 150, 782-786, 1987.

Dalton, K., *Depression After Childbirth*, Oxford University Press, Oxford, 1980.

Davidson, J.; Robertson, E., "A Follow-up of Post Partum Illness, 1946-1978," *Acta Psychiatrica Scandinavia*, Vol. 71, 451-457, 1985.

Dawson, G. et al., "Social Influences on Early Developing Biological and Behavioral Systems Related to Risk for Affective Disorder," *Development and Psychopathology*, Cambridge University Press, 1994.

DelliQuadri, L.; Breckenridge, K., *The New Mother Care*, Tarcher, Inc., Los Angeles, 1974.

Dimitrovsky, L. et al., "Depression During and Following Pregnancy: Quality of Family Relationships," *The Journal of Psychology*, Vol. 121, No. 3., 213-218, May 1987.

Eberlein, T., "Speaking with the Outspoken Penelope Leach," *New Baby*, Vol. LIV, No. 1, Jan. 1992.

Elkin, I. et al., "National Institute of Mental Health Treatment of Depression Collaborative Research Project," *Arch. General Psychiatry*, Vol. 46, Nov. 1989.

Findlay, S., "The Revolution in Psychiatric Care," *U.S. News and World Report*, Aug. 5, 1991.

Fink, G.; Sumner, B., "Estrogen and Mental State," *Nature*, Vol. 383, Sept. 26, 1996.

Fischer, L., *Linked Lives: Adult Daughters and Their Mothers*, Harper & Row, New York, 1986.

Gerstein, H.C., "How Common Is Postpartum Thyroiditis? A Methodologic Overview of the Literature," *Arch. Internal Medicine*, Vol. 150, July 1990.

Gitlin, M.; Pasnau, R., "Psychiatric Syndromes Linked to Reproductive Function in Women: A Review of Current Knowledge," *American Journal of Psychiatry*, Vol. 146, No. 11, Nov. 1989.

Gjerdingen, D.K. et al., "Changes in Women's Physical Health During the First Postpartum Year," *Archives of Family Medicine*, Vol. 2, March 1993.

Goldstein, R.L., "The Psychiatrist's Guide to Right and Wrong: Part III: Postpartum Depression and the 'Appreciation' of Wrongfulness," *Bulletin American Academy Psychiatric Law*, Vol. 17, No. 2, 1989.

Goleman, D., "Wide Beliefs on Depression in Women Contradicted," *New York Times*, Jan. 9, 1990.

Goleman, D., "Women's Depression Rate Is Higher," *New York Times*, Dec. 6, 1990.

Gordon, R. et al., "Factors in Postpartum Emotional Adjustment," *Obstetrics and Gynecology*, Vol. 25, No. 2, Feb. 1965.

Greenberg, M., *The Birth of a Father*, Avon Books, New York, 1985.

Gruen, D., *Babies and Jobs: Concerns and Choices*, Pennypress, Inc., Seattle, 1986.

Gruen, D., *The New Parent: A Spectrum of Postpartum Adjustment*, Pennypress, Inc., Seattle, 1988.

Gruen, D., "Postpartum Depression: A Debilitating Yet Often Unassessed Problem," National Association of Social Workers, Inc., *Health and Social Work*, Vol. 15, No. 4, Nov. 1990.

Hamilton, J.A., *Postpartum Psychiatric Problems*, The C.V. Mosby Co., St. Louis, 1962.

Hamilton, J.; Harberger, P.N., *Postpartum Psychiatric Illness: A Picture Puzzle*, University of Pennsylvania Press, Philadelphia, 1992.

Handford, P., "Postpartum Depression: What Is It? What Helps?" *The Canadian Nurse*, Jan. 1985.

Hapgood, C. et al., "Maternity Blues: Phenomena and Relationship to Later Post Partum Depression," *Australian and New Zealand Journal of Psychiatry*, Vol. 22, No. 3, Sept. 1988.

Harris, B. et al., "Transient Post-partum Thyroid Dysfunction and Postnatal Depression," *Journal of Affective Disorders*, Vol. 17, 243-249, 1989.

Harris, Irving B., "New Knowledge About the Human Brain and Its Meaning for Early Childhood Development," Helen Harris Perlman Lecture, May 31, 1996.

Japenga, A., "Ordeal of Postpartum Psychosis: Illness Can Have Tragic Consequences for New Mothers," *Los Angeles Times*, Feb. 1, 1987, Part VI.

Jordon, J.; Kaplan, A.; Miller, J.M.; Stiver, I.; Surrey, J., *Women's Growth in Connection*, Guilford Press, New York, 1991.

Jovanovic, L.; Subak-Sharpe, J., *Hormones: The Women's Answerbook*, Atheneum, New York, 1987.

Kalmus, D. et al., "Parenting Expectations, Experiences, and Adjustment to Parenthood: A Test of the Violated Expectations Framework," *Journal of Marriage and the Family*, Vol. 54, 519, 1992.

Kendall, R.; Chalmers, J.; Platz, C., "Epidemiology of Puerperal Psychoses," *British Journal of Psychiatry*, Vol. 150, 662-673, 1987.

Kendall, R. et al., "Mood Changes in the First Three Weeks After Childbirth," *Journal of Affective Disorders*, Vol. 3, 317-326, 1981.

Kendall, R. et al., "The Social and Obstetric Correlates of Psychiatric Admission in the Puerperium," *Psychological Medicine*, Vol. 11, 341-350, 1981.

Killien, M., *Psychosocial Influences on Postpartum Fatigue*, University of Washington, Seattle.

Kinard, E.M., "Mother and Teacher Assessments of Behavior Problems in Abused Children," *Journal of the American Academy of Child and Adolescent Psychiatry*, Vol. 34, No. 8, 1043-1053, 1995.

Kitzinger, S., *Women as Mothers*, Martin Robinson Co. Ltd., London, 1978.

Kraus, M.; Redman, E.S., "Postpartum Depression: An Interactional View," *Journal of Marital and Family Therapy*, Vol. 12, No. 1, 63-74, 1986.

Kumar, R.; Robson, K.M., "A Prospective Study of Emotional Disorders in Childbearing Women," *British Journal of Psychiatry*, Vol. 144, 35-47, 1984.

Levy, V., "The Maternity Blues in Post-partum and Post-operative Women," *British Journal of Psychiatry*, Vol. 151, 368-372, 1987.

Levy-Shiff, R., "Individual and Contextual Correlates of Marital Change Across the Transition to Parenthood," *Developmental Psychology*, Vol. 30, No. 4, 591-601, 1994.

Logan, R., "Helping a Spouse Over a Major Depression," *Medical Aspects of Human Sexuality*, May 1988.

McBride, A.B., "Mental Health Effects of Women's Multiple Roles," *American Psychologist*, Vol. 45, No. 3, 381-384, March 1990.

McGrath, E., *When Feeling Bad Is Good*, Bantam Books, New York, 1992.

McGrath, E.; Keita, G.P.; Strickland, B.; Russo, N.F., *Women and Depression*, American Psychological Association, Washington, DC, 1990.

Meltzer, E.S.; Kumar, R., "Puerperal Mental Illness, Clinical Features and Classification: A Study of 142 Mother-and-Baby Admissions," *British Journal of Psychiatry*, Vol. 147, 647-654, 1985.

Metz, A.; Sichel, D.; Goff, D., "Postpartum Panic Disorder," *Journal of Clinical Psychiatry*, Vol. 49, No. 7, July 1988.

Morris, J.B., "Group Psychotherapy for Prolonged Postnatal Depression," *British Journal of Medical Psychology*, Vol. 60, 279-281, 1987.

Morris, N., "Insanity Defense," National Institute of Justice Crime File Study Guide, U.S. Dept. of Justice.

Moss, D., "Postpartum Psychosis Defense," *American Bar Association Journal*, Vol. 74, Aug. 1, 1988.

The National Institutes of Health, "Electro-convulsive Therapy," *Consensus Development Conference Statement*, Vol. 5, No. 11.

Nott, P.M. et al., "Hormonal Changes and Mood in the Puerperium," *British Journal of Psychiatry*, Vol. 128, 379-383, 1976.

O'Hara, M., "Social Support, Life Events, and Depression During Pregnancy and the Puerperium," *Archives of General Psychiatry*, Vol. 43, June 1986.

O'Hara M. et al., "Prospective Study of Postpartum Blues: Biologic and Psychosocial Factors," *Archives of General Psychiatry*, Vol. 48, Sept. 1991.

Orr, S. et al., "Chronic Stressors and Maternal Depression: Implications for Prevention," *American Journal of Public Health*, Vol. 79, No. 9, Sept. 1989.

Osofsky, H., "Efficacious Treatments of PMS: A Need for Further Research," *Journal of the American Medical Association*, Vol. 264, No. 3, July 18, 1990.

Pacific Post Partum Support Society, "Post Partum Depression and Anxiety," Vancouver, B.C., 1987.

Parry, B., "Mood Disorders Linked to the Reproductive Cycle in Women," from *Psychopharmacology: The Fourth General of Progress*, Bloom, F., and Kupfer, D., eds., Raven Press, Ltd., New York, 1995.

Paykel, E. et al., "Life Events and Social Support in Puerperal Depression," *British Journal of Psychiatry*, Vol. 136, 339-346, 1980.

Pop, V., "Postpartum Thyroid Dysfunction and Depression in an Unselected Population," *New England Journal of Medicine*, Vol. 324, No. 25, June 20, 1991.

Price, J., *Motherhood: What It Does to Your Mind*, Pandora, London, 1989.

Quadagno, D. et al., "Postpartum Moods in Men and Women," *American Journal of Obstetrics and Gynecology*, Vol. 154, No. 5, May 1986.

Ramsay, I., "Postpartum Thyroiditis — An Underdiagnosed Disease," *British Journal of Obstetrics and Gynaecology*, Vol. 93, 1121-1123, Nov. 1986.

Regier, D., "The NIMH Depression Awareness, Recognition, and Treatment Program: Structure, Aims, and Scientific Basis," *American Journal of Psychiatry*, Vol. 145, No. 11, Nov. 1988.

Robson, K.M.; Kumar, R., "Delayed Onset of Maternal Affection After Childbirth," *British Journal of Psychiatry*, Vol. 136, 347-353, 1980.

Rosenberg, H., "Motherwork, Stress and Depression: The Costs of Privatized Social Reproduction," *Feminism and Political Economy: Women's Work, Women's Struggles*, Ch. 10, Methuen, 1987.

Rosenthal, N.; Wehr, T., "Seasonal Affective Disorder," *Psychiatric Annals*, Vol. 17, Oct. 10, 1987.

Russell, D., "Postpartum Insanity: A Troubling Defense," *The Legal Intelligencer*, Vol. 200, No. 33, Feb. 21, 1989.

Schopf, J. et al., "A Family Hereditary Study of Post-partum 'Psychosis,'" *European Archives of Psychiatric Neurological Science*, Vol. 235, 164-170, 1985.

Silverstein, L., "Transforming the Debate About Child Care and Maternal Employment," *American Psychologist*, Vol. 46, No. 10, 1025-1032, Oct. 1991.

Sosa, R. et al., "The Effect of a Supportive Companion on Perinatal Problems, Length of Labor, and Mother-Infant Interaction," *New England Journal of Medicine*, Vol. 303, No. 11, Sept. 11, 1980.

Stein, R., "Marriage, Poverty, Abuse Tied to Women's Depression," United Press International, Dec. 5, 1990.

Stoddard, A., *Mothers: A Celebration*, William Morrow & Co., New York, 1996.

Stuart, S., "Treatment of Postpartum Depression with Interpersonal Psychotherapy," *Archives of General Psychiatry*, Vol. 52, Jan. 1995.

Susan, V.; Katz, J., "Weaning and Depression: Another Postpartum Complication," *American Journal of Psychiatry*, Vol. 145, No. 4, April 1988.

Swigart, J., *The Myth of the Bad Mother*, Doubleday, New York, 1991.

Taubman, B., *Curing Infant Colic: The 7-Minute Program for Soothing the Fussy Baby*, Bantam Books, New York, 1990.

Tentoni, S.; High, K., "Culturally Induced Postpartum Depression: A Theoretical Position," *JOGN*, Vol. 9, No. 4, July/August 1990.

Thomas, P., "Depression: Younger Patients, Newer Therapies," *Medical World News*, Aug. 1990.

Ungar, J., "'Good' Mothers Feel Dark Urges," *New York Times*, May 10, 1988.

U.S. Department of Health and Human Services, "Depression: What You Need to Know," DHHS Publication No. 87-1543, 1987.

U.S. Department of Health and Human Services, "Depressive Illnesses: Treatments Bring New Hope," DHHS Publication No. 89-1491, 1986/1989.

U.S. Department of Labor, Bureau of Labor Statistics, "Employee Benefits in Medium and Large Firms, 1989," June 1990.

Watson, J. et al., "Psychiatric Disorder in Pregnancy and the First Postnatal Year," *British Journal of Psychiatry*, Vol. 144, 453-462, 1984.

Weissman, M.; Prusoff, B.A.; Dimascio, A. et al., "The Efficacy of Drugs and Psychotherapy in the Treatment of Acute Depressive Disorders," *American Journal of Psychiatry*, Vol. 136, 555-558.

Wells, K. et al., "The Functioning and Well-being of Depressed Patients: Results from the Medical Outcomes Study," *Journal of the American Medical Association*, Vol. 262, No. 7, Aug. 18, 1989.

Whiffen, V., "Screening for Postpartum Depression: A Methodological Note," *Journal of Clinical Psychology*, Vol. 44, No. 3, May 1988.

Wrate, R. et al., "Postnatal Depression and Child Development: A Three-Year Follow-up Study," *British Journal of Psychiatry*, Vol. 146, 622-627, 1985.

Yalom, I. et al., "Postpartum Blues Syndrome: A Description and Related Variables," *Archives of General Psychiatry*, Vol. 18, Jan. 1968.

Yen, M., "High-risk Mothers: Postpartum Depression, in Rare Cases, May Trigger Infanticide," *Washington Post*, Aug. 23, 1988.

Zuckerman, B.; Beardslee, W., "Maternal Depression: A Concern for Pediatricians," *Pediatrics*, Vol. 79, No. 1, Jan. 1987.

Endnotes

Chapter One

1. Sichel, D., "Comprehensive Treatment Planning: Biological Approaches," Remarks from the Fifth Annual Conference of Postpartum Support International, Pittsburgh, PA, 1991.

2. Kendell, R.E., "Suicide in Pregnancy and the Puerperium," *British Medical Journal*, Vol. 302, p. 126-127.

3. Hines, C., "Psychiatric Illness in the Postpartum Period," Remarks from the Fourth Annual Conference of Postpartum Support International, St. Louis, MO, 1990.

4. Wells, K., et al., "The Functioning and Well-being of Depressed Patients: Results From the Medical Outcomes Study," *Journal of the American Medical Association*, Vol. 262, No. 7, Aug. 18, 1989.

5. "Helpful Facts About Depressive Illnesses," U.S. Department of Health and Human Services, DHHS Publication No. 89-1536. 1987/89.

6. Yalom, I., et al., " 'Postpartum Blues' Syndrome: A Description and Related Variables," *Archives of General Psychiatry*, Vol. 18, January 1968.

7. Quadagno, D., et al., "Postpartum Moods in Men and Women," *American Journal of Obstetrics and Gynecology*, Vol. 154, No. 5, May 1986.

8. Pitt, B., "Atypical Depression Following Childbirth," *British Journal of Psychiatry*, Vol. 114, 1968.

Chapter Two

1. Parry, B., "Mood Disorders Linked to Reproductive Cycle in Women," from *Psychopharmacology: The Fourth Generation of Progress*, Bloom, F., Kupfer, D., eds., Raven Press, Ltd., New York, 1995.

2. Hines, C., "Psychiatric Illness in the Postpartum Period," Remarks from the Fourth Annual Conference of Postpartum Support International, St. Louis, MO, 1990.

Chapter Three

1. Kalmuss, D., "Parenting Expectations, Experiences, and Adjustment to Parenthood: A Test of the Violated Expectations Framework," *Journal of Marriage and the Family*, Vol. 54, 1992.

2. Tulman, L.; Fawcett, J., "Recovery from Childbirth: Looking Back 6 Months After Delivery," *Health Care Women Int.*, Vol. 12, 1991.

3. Tentoni, S.; High, K., "Culturally Induced Postpartum Depression," *JOGN Nursing*, Vol. 9, No. 4, 1980.

Chapter Four

1. Harkness, S., "The Cultural Mediation of Postpartum Depression," *Medical Anthropology Quarterly*, Vol. 1, No. 2, June 1967.

2. Cosminksy, S., "Childbirth and Midwifery on a Guatemalan Finca,'" *Medical Anthropology*, Vol. 1, p. 69-104, 1977.

3. Tentoni, S.; High, K., "Culturally Induced Postpartum Depression: A Theoretical Position," *JOGN Nursing*, Vol. 9, No. 4, July-August 1980.

4. McGrat, et al., *Women and Depression*, American Psychological Assn., Washington, DC, 1990.

5. Gutloff, K., "Hard Times," *Services Employees Union*, Vol. 5, No. 2, Spring 1991.

6. Richter, P.; Martinez G., "Clinton Signs Family Leave Bill Into Law," *Los Angeles Times*, Feb. 6, 1993.

Chapter Five

1. Meltzer, E.; Kumar, R., "Puerperal Mental Illness, Clinical Features and Classification: A Study of 142 Mother-and-Baby Admissions," *British Journal of Psychiatry*, Vol. 147, 1985.

2. Institute for Bio-Behavioral Therapy and Research, "Onset of Obsessive-Compulsive Disorder in Pregnancy," *American Journal of Psychiatry*, July 1992.

3. Kumar, R., Robson, K., "Neurotic Disturbance During Pregnancy and the Puerperium: Preliminary Report of a Prospective Survey of 119 Primiparae," *Mental Illness in Pregnancy and the Puerperium*, Oxford Medical Publications, 1978.

4. "Review of Research Finds Abortion Does Not Pose Psychological Hazard for Most Women," *University of Buffalo News*, April 5, 1990.

5. Neugebauer, R., "Communication Can Lift Miscarriage Depression," *American Journal of Obstetrics and Gynecology*, Vol. 166, p. 104-109.

6. Cox, J.L, et al., "Prospective Study of the Psychiatric Disorders of Childbirth," *British Journal of Psychiatry*, Vol. 140, p. 111-117, 1982.

7. Kennerley, H.; Gath, D., "Maternity Blues, III: Associations with Obstetric, Psychological, and Psychiatric Factors," *British Journal of Psychiatry*, Vol. 155, p. 367-373, 1989.

8. Sosa, R., "The Effect of a Supportive Companion on Perinatal Problems, Length of Labor, and Mother-Infant Interaction," *The New England Journal of Medicine*, Vol. 303, No. 11, Sept. 11, 1980.

9. O'Hara, M., et al., "Prospective Study of Postpartum Blues: Biological and Psychosocial Factors," *Archives of General Psychiatry*, Vol. 48, September 1991.

10. "Physicians Not Prepared to Counsel Breast Feeding Mothers, Study Finds," NICHD News Notes, U.S. Department of Health and Human Services.

11. Van, J., Kotulak, R., "Risk of Postpartum Fatigue, Depression Highest 2 Weeks After Delivery," *Chicago Tribune*, July 8, 1990.

12. Ross, C., et al., "Dividing Work, Sharing Work, and In-between: Marriage Patterns and Depression," *American Sociological Review*, Vol. 48, p. 809-823.

13. Watson, J., et al., "Psychiatric Disorder in Pregnancy and the First Postnatal Year," *British Journal of Psychiatry*, Vol. 144, p. 453-462, 1984.

14. McGrath, E., "National Task Force on Women and Depression News Conference," *American Psychological Assn.*, Washington, DC, Dec. 5, 1990.

Chapter Six

1. Jovanovic, L.; Subak-Sharpe, G., *Hormones: The Women's Answer Book*, Atheneum, New York, 1987.

2. Kuevi, V., et al., "Plasma Amine and Hormone Changes in 'Postpartum Blues.'" *Clinical Endocrinology*, Vol. 19, p. 39-46, 1983.

3. Nott, P., et al., "Hormonal Changes and Mood in the Puerperium," *British Journal of Psychiatry*, Vo. 128, p. 379-383, 1976.

4. Parry, B., "Mood Disorders Linked to Reproductive Cycle in Women," from *Psychopharmacology: The Fourth Generation of Progress*, Bloom, F., Kupfer, D., eds., Raven Press, Ltd., New York, 1995.

5. Ramsay, I., "Commentary: Postpartum Thyroiditis — an Underdiagnosed Disease." *British Journal of Obstetrics and Gynaecology*, Vol. 93, p. 1121-1123, November 1986.

6. Ramsay, I., "Commentary: Postpartum Thyroiditis — an Underdiagnosed Disease," *British Journal of Obstetrics and Gynaecology*, Vol. 93, p. 1121-1123, November 1986.

7. Fink, G.; Sumner, B., "Estrogen and Mental State," *Nature*, Vol. 383, Sept. 26, 1996.

8. Susman, V.; Katz, J., "Weaning and Depression: Another Postpartum Complication," *American Journal of Psychiatry*, Vol. 145, No. 4, April 1988.

Chapter Seven

1. McGrath, et al., Women and Depression, American Psychological Assn., Washington, DC, 1990.

2. Mintz, L., Survey of psychology interns, University of Southern California, 1990.

3. Conley, B., remarks at the Fifth Annual Conference of Postpartum Support International, Pittsburgh, PA, 1991.

4. Weissman, M., et al., "Depressed Outpatients: Results One Year After Treatment with Drugs and/or Interpersonal Psychotherapy," *Archives of General Psychiatry*, Vol. 36, p. 51-55, 1981.

5. Sacco, W.P.; Beck, A.T., "Cognitive Theory of Depression," *Handbook of Depression: Treatment, Assessment, and Research*, Beckham, E., Leber, W., eds., Dorsey Press, Homewood, IL, 1985.

6. Stuart, S., "Treatment of Postpartum Depression with Interpersonal Psychotherapy," *Archives of General Psychiatry*, Vol. 52, January 1995.

7. McGrath, et al., Women and Depression, American Psychological Association, Washington, DC, 1990.

Chapter Eight

1. Kraus, M.; Redman, S., "Postpartum Depression: An Interactional View," *Journal of Marital and Family Therapy*, Vol. 12, No. 1, January 1986.

2. Gordon, R., et al., "Factors in Postpartum Emotional Adjustment," *Obstetrics & Gynecology*, Vol. 25, p. 158-166, February, 1965.

3. Pacific Post Partum Support Society, "Post Partum Anxiety and Depression," Vancouver, BC, 1987.

4. Pacific Post Partum Support Society, "Post Partum Anxiety and Depression," Vancouver, BC, 1987.

5. Pacific Post Partum Support Society, "Post Partum Anxiety and Depression," Vancouver, BC, 1987.

6. Pacific Post Partum Support Society, "Post Partum Anxiety and Depression," Vancouver, BC, 1987.

7. Pacific Post Partum Support Society, "Post Partum Anxiety and Depression," Vancouver, BC, 1987.

8. McGrath, et al., Women and Depression, American Psychological Association, Washington, DC, 1990.

Chapter Nine

1. Atkinson, A.; Rickel, A., "Postpartum Depression in Primaparous Parents," *Journal of Abnormal Psychology*, Vol. 93, p. 115-119, 1984.

2. Zaslow, M., et al., "Depressed Mood in New Fathers: Interview and Behavior Correlates," Boston: Society for Research in Child Development, 1981.

3. Tronick, E., Remarks at "Depression During Pregnancy and the Postpartum Period" conference, Newton-Wellesley Hospital, May 2, 1991.

4. Kumar, R.; Robson, K., "A Prospective Study of Emotional Disorders in Childbearing Women," *British Journal of Psychiatry*, Vol. 144, p. 35-47, 1984.

5. Kumar, R.; Robson, K., "Delayed Onset of Maternal Affection After Childbirth," *British Journal of Psychiatry*, Vol. 136, p. 347-353, 1980.

6. Ainsworth, M.D.S., et al., "Patterns of Infant Attachment," Erlbaum: Hillsdale, NJ, 1978.

7. Coghill, S.R., et al., "Impact of Maternal Postnatal Depression on Cognitive Development of Young Children," *British Medical Journal*, Vol. 292, p. 1165-1167, 1986.

8. Research by Field, T., University of Miami, From paper to the American Psychological Association. Reported in: "Depressive Aftermath for New Mothers," *Science News*, Vol. 138.

9. The Commonwealth Fund, "The Commonwealth Fund Survey of Parents with Young Children," August 1996.

10. Research by Jeffrey Cohn, University of Pittsburgh, From paper to the American Psychological Association, Reported in: "Depressive Aftermath for New Mothers," *Science News*, Vol. 138.

11. Kinard, E.M., "Mother and Teacher Assessments of Behavior Problems in Abused Children," *Journal of the American Academy of Child and Adolescent Psychiatry*, Vol. 34, No. 8, 1043-1053, 1995.

12. The Commonwealth Fund, "The Commonwealth Fund Survey of Parents with Young Children," August 1996.

13. Quinton, D.; Rutter, M., "Family Pathology and Child Psychiatric Disorder: A Four Year Prospective Study," *Longitudinal Studies in Child Psychology and Psychiatry: Practical Lessons for Research Experience*, Nichol, A.R., ed., Wiley: Chichester, England, 1985.

14. Weissman, M., et al., "Children of Depressed Parents: Increased Psychopathology and Early Onset of Major Depression," *Archives of General Psychiatry*, Vol. 44, p. 847-863, 1987.

Chapter Ten

1. Gordon, R., et al., "Factors in Postpartum Emotional Adjustment," *Obstetrics & Gynecology*, Vol. 25, p. 158-166, February, 1965.

2. Gordon, R., et al., "Factors in Postpartum Emotional Adjustment," *Obstetrics & Gynecology*, Vol. 25, p. 158-166, February, 1965.

3. Gordon, R., et al., "Factors in Postpartum Emotional Adjustment," *Obstetrics & Gynecology*, Vol. 25, No. 2, February, 1965.

Index